Praise for *Choose Life*

Choose Life is a thorough and articulate examination of the pro-life position by multiple highly qualified contributors. Their challenges to the pro-choice position are reasoned and thoughtful. Whether you're pro-life, pro-choice, or on the fence, this book has much to offer you.

Randy Alcorn
Bestselling author of *Why Pro-Life?*, *ProLife Answers to ProChoice Arguments*, and *Pro-Choice or Pro-Life?*

Addressing theological, philosophical, legal, spiritual, and practical concerns, the contributors not only do not shy away from the difficult questions, but answer them with intelligence, care, and compassion. I can't think of another book with such breadth and depth that is also accessible to ordinary people who want to learn more about what it truly means to choose life.

Francis J. Beckwith
Professor of Philosophy & Church-State Studies, and Affiliate Professor of Political Science, Baylor University

The defense of human dignity and the sanctity of human life is one of the central and inescapable tasks of today's Christians. In that task, we need every hand on deck. In *Choose Life*, a first-rank team of Christian defenders of life addresses some of the most pressing questions of our day, and with conviction they counter some of the most influential arguments coming from abortion supporters. This book is timely—urgently so—and will be a great encouragement to Christians in the battle for life.

R. Albert Mohler Jr.
President, The Southern Baptist Theological Seminary

Choose Life is at once both informative and inspiring. The diverse backgrounds of the contributors give the book an impressive breadth and balance—biblical scholarship, philosophical reasoning, legal analysis, public policy, biology, medicine, counseling, personal reflection from experience—*Choose Life* has something for everyone! This book is a helpful resource that can be used both to equip and to persuade.

Benjamin Wilson
Lead Pastor, Harvest Bible Chapel, Fayetteville, AR

Abortion is more than a political, cultural, hot-button topic. A Christian must meet this issue with biblical wisdom, an empathetic understanding of women's circumstances followed by considerable solutions. *Choose Life* gives a voice to the unborn and will direct life-giving, healing conversations.

Candace Cameron Bure
Actress, producer, author, mother of three

On any number of occasions, Black pastors, tired of the news they're getting from the mainstream media, have reached out to me regarding the pro-life movement's leadership, mission, and heart. This book addresses all of those critically important issues and much, much more.

Walter B. Hoye II
Pro-life leader of Issues4Life Foundation

This is simply a splendid collection of essays. Every pro-lifer who wants to bear witness to the truth about the profound dignity of every human being and our obligations to support women as they bear new life will benefit from this book. No one can afford to sit on the sidelines, and *Choose Life* will help you defend life.

Ryan T. Anderson
President of the Ethics and Public Policy Center

Choose Life is the most thorough work on answering objections in recent years. The up-to-date material found in these pages has been painstakingly researched by some of the brightest and most caring minds on the subject and will be a training manual for any serious student for years to come. I enthusiastically recommend this book to anyone who would like to research the pro-life position with integrity. Any desire of mine to write on this sensitive subject was dispelled as I realized *everything* I've ever wanted to say was lovingly covered. You will cry and you will rejoice as intimate stories of courage, betrayal, and hope are on full display for your consideration to choose life.
Ray Comfort
Founder and CEO of Living Waters ministries and the bestselling author of more than 90 books

If ever there were an issue that needs to be approached with grace, truth, and compassion, it is abortion in America. This book has done it. Tens of millions of our neighbors' lives have been lost or devastated through abortion since *Roe v. Wade* mandated abortion-on-demand in our country and ignited a bitter national debate that continues to this day. *Choose Life* gives us a comprehensive framework for approaching this ongoing tragedy with resolve, and with specific action steps to love the human beings involved.
Denise Harle
Sr. Counsel, Alliance Defending Freedom; former Deputy Solicitor General of Florida; board member of a women's pregnancy center

Jeanette Hagen Pifer and John K. Goodrich have done us the wonderful service of bringing together an outstanding collection of essays that address a vitally important theme. *Choose Life* delivers admirably on its subtitle's promise. Leading scholars from a range of disciplines answer the most pressing claims of abortion defenders—and do so with clarity, courage, and importantly, compassion. An excellent resource!
Todd Wilson
Cofounder and President, The Center for Pastor Theologians

Choose Life is a thorough and sensitive look at abortion and the discussion between pro-choice and pro-life advocates. It considers the topic from every angle—philosophical, theological, legal, social, cultural, and, most importantly, from the standpoint of a woman's long-term experience. It drips with a sensitive tone, often lacking in this conversation. This book explains why being pro-life promotes our overall social well-being and deep care for the woman who faces a challenging, life-altering, deeply moral choice.

Darrell L. Bock
Executive Director for Cultural Engagement, the Howard G. Hendricks Center for Christian Leadership and Cultural Engagement; Senior Research Professor of New Testament Studies, Dallas Theological Seminary

CHOOSE LIFE

ANSWERING KEY CLAIMS *of* ABORTION DEFENDERS *with* COMPASSION

GENERAL EDITORS

JEANETTE HAGEN PIFER
and JOHN K. GOODRICH

Moody Publishers
CHICAGO

Some content in chapter 4 is adapted from Scott B. Rae and Paul M. Cox, Bioethics: *A Christian Approach in a Pluralistic Age* (Grand Rapids: Eerdmans, 1999) and Scott B. Rae, *Moral Choices: An Introduction to Ethics* (Grand Rapids: Zondervan, 2009).

Personal stories have been shared with permission, though some names and details may have been changed to protect privacy. All resources listed are accurate at the time of publication but may change in the future.

Edited by Pamela J. Pugh
Interior design: Ragont Design
Cover design: Charles Brock
Cover illustration of leaves copyright © 2020 by pashabo / Vector Stock (941678).
Cover illustration of mountains copyright © 2020 by Vitalez / Adobe Stock (300729038).
Cover illustration of watercolor copyright © 2020 by Abbies Art Shop / Adobe Stock (298359661).
Cover photo of paper texture copyright © 2014 by DNKSTUDIO/ Depositphotos (54093345).
Cover illustration of brush strokes copyright © 2016 by aga77ta/ Depositphotos (123531452).
All rights reserved for all of the above backgrounds/textures.
Author photo of Jeanette Hagen Pifer: Marissa Lundy
Author photo of John Goodrich: courtesy of Moody Bible Institute

Photo credits: Amy Ford: Meshali Mitchell; Tara Sander Lee: courtesy of the *Milwaukee Business Journal*; Charlotte Pence: Amelia Cassar Photography; Joy Riley: Ian Riley

Library of Congress Cataloging-in-Publication Data

Names: Hagen Pifer, Jeanette, editor. | Goodrich, John K., editor.
Title: Choose life : answering key claims of abortion defenders with compassion / Jeanette Hagen Pifer, editor and John K. Goodrich, editor.
Description: Chicago : Moody Publishers, 2022. | Includes bibliographical references. | Summary: "Choose Life provides pro-life responses from leading experts who help you know what to say-and why to say it-when you're faced with pro-abortion claims. No more fist-shaking and hurled insults. Learn to make the pro-life case with intelligent arguments and compassionate love-just the way a Christian should"-- Provided by publisher.
Identifiers: LCCN 2021033787 (print) | LCCN 2021033788 (ebook) | ISBN 9780802421739 (paperback) | ISBN 9780802499257 (ebook)
Subjects: LCSH: Abortion--Religious aspects--Christianity. | Pro-life movement.
Classification: LCC HQ767.25 .C49 2022 (print) | LCC HQ767.25 (ebook) | DDC 241/.6976--dc23
LC record available at https://lccn.loc.gov/2021033787
LC ebook record available at https://lccn.loc.gov/2021033788

Originally delivered by fleets of horse-drawn wagons, the affordable paperbacks from D. L. Moody's publishing house resourced the church and served everyday people. Now, after more than 125 years of publishing and ministry, Moody Publishers' mission remains the same—even if our delivery systems have changed a bit. For more information on other books and resources created from a biblical perspective, go to www.moodypublishers.com or write to:

Moody Publishers
820 N. LaSalle Boulevard
Chicago, IL 60610

1 3 5 7 9 10 8 6 4 2

Printed in the United States of America

For our sons,

Justin Dylan Goodrich

and

Brantley John Pifer

"Behold, children are a heritage from the LORD,
the fruit of the womb a reward."
Psalm 127:3

Contents

Contributors

EDITORS

John K. Goodrich, PhD, is Professor of Bible at Moody Bible Institute and is author or editor of several academic books and articles. He recently published *Following Jesus Christ: The New Testament Message of Discipleship for Today*. His PhD is in New Testament studies from Durham University.

Jeanette Hagen Pifer, PhD, is Assistant Professor of New Testament at Talbot School of Theology, Biola University. She is author or editor of several books and articles. Jeanette has served in a variety of ministry capacities, including evangelistic and humanitarian work with orphans in the former Soviet Union, and in the facilitation of theological education around the world. Her PhD is in New Testament studies from Durham University.

* * * * * * *

Christina Bennett is Director of Communications at the Family Institute of Connecticut. Christina is a foster parent and has served as a pro-life advocate, a missionary, and the Client Services Manager for a Pregnancy Resource Center in her home state of Connecticut.

Bethany Bomberger is a speaker, activist, adoptive mother, and the Executive Director of the Radiance Foundation, which she co-founded with her husband, Ryan. She is the author of the children's book *Pro-Life Kids!*

Charlotte Pence Bond is a bestselling author and the daughter of former Vice President Mike Pence. Her work has been published or featured in the *Washington Times, Glamour* magazine, *US Weekly,* and other major media outlets. A graduate of DePaul University with a degree in Digital Cinema Screenwriting and English, Charlotte contributed to the Emmy Award–winning documentary *Fleeced.* A pro-life activist and speaker, Charlotte recently received her Master of Theological Studies degree from Harvard Divinity School. She currently works as a writer and reporter at *The Daily Wire.*

Sandy Christiansen, MD, is a board-certified obstetrician/gynecologist and advocate for the sanctity of human life from conception to natural death. She is the National Medical Director for Care Net, one of the largest networks of pregnancy centers in North America. Locally, she is the Medical Director for the Care Net Pregnancy Center of Frederick, MD, and an adjunct professor at Mount St. Mary's University, where she teaches healthcare policy at the graduate level. Sandy is a writer and speaker on pregnancy, abortion, and Hippocratic medicine, addressing a variety of forums including the United Nations, the President's Council on Bioethics, and various legislative bodies. She also provides commentary to national media outlets. Her medical degree is from the Medical College of Pennsylvania.

Josh J. Craddock, JD, is an affiliated scholar with the James Wilson Institute. He is a graduate of the Harvard Law School, where he served as editor in chief of the *Harvard Journal of Law & Public Policy*. He later clerked for the Honorable Chief Judge Timothy Tymkovich of the US Court of Appeals for the Tenth District. Prior to law school, Josh managed advocacy teams for several nonprofit organizations at the United Nations. His writing has appeared in the *Notre Dame Law Review*, the *Harvard Journal on Legislation, First Things, Newsweek*, and *National Review*.

Catherine Davis is the Founder and President of the Restoration Project, which is dedicated to rebuilding families, promoting the sanctity of life, and providing related educational materials, in order to transform American public policy and culture's impact on Black life into a restored culture of uprightness, evenhandedness, and virtue. Catherine is author of *The Fight for Life: Taking It to the Street* and *The Fight for Life: Turning the Wounded into Warriors*. She attended the University of Bridgeport School of Law, and now serves on the advisory board to Human Coalition and Day of Tears, and on the Spera Vita Institute Advocacy Council.

Carlynn Fabarez is a Bible teacher and the wife of Pastor Mike Fabarez, the Senior Pastor of Compass Bible Church and host of Focal Point Radio. She and Mike have been married and working together in the local church for over three decades. They are parents of three grown children, including Stephanie, who was prenatally diagnosed with a serious disability.

Amy Ford is cofounder and President of Embrace Grace, a nonprofit that inspires and equips the church to love on single and pregnant young women and their families. She is also the author of *Help Her Be Brave: Discover Your Place in the Pro-Life Movement.* Amy speaks nationally to varied audiences including women's ministry events, pro-life and adoption conferences, church leadership equipping, and pregnancy center benefits.

Catherine Glenn Foster, MA, JD, is President and CEO of Americans United for Life, America's original national pro-life organization and the nation's premier pro-life legal team. Catherine has authored, testified on, and litigated numerous domestic, foreign, and international legislation and initiatives. She has also testified before and advised the US Senate Judiciary Committee, the US House of Representatives Committee on Energy and Commerce Select Investigative Panel and its Subcommittee on Oversight and Investigations, and other federal and state bodies and representatives. Catherine earned her law degree from Georgetown University Law Center.

Donna Harrison, MD, is a board-certified obstetrician/gynecologist and the Executive Director of the American Association of Prolife Obstetricians and Gynecologists, the largest pro-life physician organization in the world. She has spoken before the FDA Reproductive Health Advisory Committee on mifepristone and ulipristal and has addressed numerous congressional committees, as well as presenting at the United Nations Committee on the Status of Women accessory sessions on topics related to medical abortion in developing nations, and maternal mortality and abortion. Her medical degree is from the University of Michigan Medical School.

Paula Ilari is the Executive Director for Hope After Rape Conception, a pro-life nonprofit dedicated to assisting mothers from rape and their children. Paula founded the ministry after she herself conceived her older son, Caleb, through gang rape. Paula's story has been featured by an assortment of international media. A devoted advocate for her son and all people conceived like him, Paula enjoys speaking at pro-life fundraisers and events to share her testimony of conversion from pro-choice volunteer with Planned Parenthood and a private abortion facility to pro-life activist.

Dr. Kendra Kolb is a practicing Neonatologist in Pennsylvania. She received her medical degree from Drexel University College of Medicine, and completed her Pediatric Residency and Neonatal-Perinatal Medicine fellowship training at St. Christophers Hospital for Children in Philadelphia, PA. She is certified by the American Board of Pediatrics in both Pediatrics and Neonatal-Perinatal Medicine. In addition to serving as an active member on the Board of Directors at a local pregnancy care center, she has been involved in the pro-life movement in a variety of capacities, including previous work with Live Action, Students for Life of America, and speaker at the 2020 National Prolife Summit. She is also a wife and proud mother of three children.

Tara Sander Lee, PhD, is the Senior Fellow and Director of Life Sciences at the Charlotte Lozier Institute, an organization dedicated to policies and practices that protect the sanctity of human life. She is a scientist with academic and clinical medicine experience in pediatric disease. She is published in medical journals and textbooks, has given expert congressional testimony, provides scientific advice for legislators and policymakers, and is a member of the US Department of Health and Human Services Secretary's Advisory Committee on Infant Mortality. Her PhD in Biochemistry is from the Medical College of Wisconsin and fellowship training in Cell and Molecular Biology from Harvard Medical School.

Patrina Mosley is a speaker and advocate for women on the issues of the right to life and combating sexual exploitation. Her commentary has been featured in the *New York Times*, the *Washington Post*, *Washington Examiner*, *The Hill*, *Townhall*, *The Federalist*, *World Magazine*, and more. She has also testified before various state legislatures and the US Senate Judiciary Committee. Patrina formerly served at United States Agency for International Development and the Family Research Council as the Director of Life, Culture, and Women's Advocacy. She is a graduate of Liberty University with a BS in Religion and a master's degree in Public Policy.

Scott B. Rae, PhD, is a prominent Christian philosopher and ethicist who serves as Dean of the Faculty and Professor of Philosophy and Christian Ethics at Talbot School of Theology, Biola University. He is a former president of the Evangelical Theological Society and is the author of numerous books and articles, including *Moral Choices: An Introduction to Ethics*, *Bioethics: A Christian Approach in a Pluralistic Age*, and *Body & Soul: Human Nature and the Crisis in Ethics*. His PhD is from the University of Southern California.

D. Joy Riley, MD, is board-certified in internal medicine and serves as Executive Director of the Tennessee Center for Bioethics & Culture. Joy is the coauthor of *Christian Bioethics: A Guide for Pastors,*

Health Care Professionals, and Families and *Outside the Womb: Moral Guidance for Assisted Reproduction* (with Scott Rae). Her medical degree is from the University of Kentucky College of Medicine, and she also has a master's degree in bioethics from Trinity International University, where she is an adjunct professor in the graduate school.

Victoria Robinson is an author, a national public speaker, and television personality. She's been a highly regarded and respected voice in the pro-life movement for almost three decades. She is the author of *They Lied to Us,* a compilation of stories from women who regretted choosing abortion. Her sequel, *They Lied to Us Too,* shares the stories of men also affected by abortion trauma. Victoria is the President and Founder of ReAssemble, a counseling ministry to post-abortive men and women. She speaks around the world in churches, youth and women's conferences, and pregnancy resource center fundraising events.

Sarah Zagorski was rescued from abortion after her immigrant birth mother was referred to a New Orleans abortionist. Although the doctor intended to leave Sarah for dead following a breech delivery at 26 weeks, her mother made a miraculous pro-life decision and successfully fought for Sarah's life. After spending her earliest years in the foster care system, Sarah was adopted at the age of nine. Today, Sarah is a wife, mother, and an advocate for life, foster care, and adoption with Louisiana Right to Life.

Foreword

—Dr. Alveda C. King—

The United States Supreme Court's *Roe v. Wade* decision in 1973 made abortion—the killing of innocent preborn baby human beings in the womb—legal in every state. For some, this decision remains a landmark civil rights victory. For others, this decision is among the most invasive of crimes against humanity, and is an atrocity against the civil rights of America's youngest and weakest victims, our babies. According to Acts 17:26, God created us all as one race, one blood. We are all brothers and sisters in Christ and should love and protect each other, from the womb to the tomb.

When the decision to legalize abortion was handed down, medical technology was not as advanced as it is today. Furthermore, at that time we did not hear public testimonies regarding the harmful impact of abortion. For not only were the babies being handed death sentences . . . the mothers too who would suffer the aftermath of abortion had yet to sing their sad songs. I know this too well—I am one of the countless women who regrets her abortions. Today, thousands of our testimonies are now on record. Our accounts are published in blogs, amicus briefs, books, songs, and films—and in the secret annals of our pain. Thankfully, there is victory beyond the pain. Today, many of us are now repentant and are raising our voices and our platforms to expose the scourge of abortion in America.

New voices and messengers are rising. The editors and contributors of *Choose Life* are among those voices and their message is clear. In this book, we have twenty essays authored by leading thinkers and activists in the fields of medicine, law, social justice, and more. Their wisdom and practical responses to defenders of abortion are there to be pondered, studied, and absorbed—with the hope, expectations, and prayers that what we learn will cause us to be part of the solution.

As we rise above merely pointing out the problems, we must seek answers. This book is a key, a guide, to finding solutions to the scourge of abortion. The messages herein offer an invaluable resource for addressing the realities of abortion, and the issues associated with them. As we read and discover the pain, anxiety, and concerns of real women—and men too—we must come to see that Christ is the answer, the solution to the problems caused by abortion.

Finally, the book will provide you as the reader with credible resources to help you answer pro-choice claims with confidence and compassion. This book is for the learned apologists and everyday thinkers alike. For too long, well-meaning Christians have been largely unprepared in defending prenatal life. It is time now to wake up, to tell the truth about abortion, and do so without fear or doubting. It is time for faith and works to come together, without compromising the witness of the gospel.

The conflict between defenders of life and proponents of death is as old as the battle between good and evil. In *Choose Life,* editors Jeanette Pifer and John Goodrich, along with their team of contributors, answer key claims of abortion defenders with both conviction and compassion.

INTRODUCTION

A Call for Compassionate Engagement

—Jeanette Hagen Pifer and John K. Goodrich—

Choose life, that you and your offspring may live.
Deuteronomy 30:19

Haunted.

This is the word many women use to describe their day-to-day experience after having an abortion. Their haunting includes fear, guilt, shame, confusion, but most of all, the memory of the life that was—and could have been.

Countless women bury these memories deep within. One woman, Elizabeth, recalls being young and poor, with two small children. As a single mom, she worked night and day just to feed her little ones. When she found herself with another positive pregnancy test, fear and insecurity welled up within her as she prepared to tell her then-boyfriend. She expected him to show support and to commit to being there, both for her and for their baby. She hoped he would marry her, that he would father her three children, and that they would live happily ever after. Instead, he rationalized: "Now is not really a good time. I think you should have an abortion." After seeing her through the procedure, he abruptly ended the relationship. She was devastated and left to mourn her losses.

Another woman, Lydia, shared her story of teenage pregnancy. Lydia's family was church-going, but not a Christ-centered household. Alcohol consumed her father, and her mother was emotionally absent, so Lydia began looking to young men for love and attention. At sixteen, she found herself pregnant, and thankfully, her son is with her today. But when she became pregnant a second, and then a third time, Lydia's mother forced her to abort. She still weeps over the loss of her beloved babies.

A third story concerns a woman at a completely different stage of life. This one is about Cynthia, who in her early thirties was seeking to live life to the fullest—at least in the way the world believes a full life ought to be lived. Finding career success by day and an exciting social life by night, Cynthia too found herself unexpectedly pregnant. Mentally unprepared to become a mother and afraid to raise a child alone, she was unsure about what to do. Heeding the popular message that abortion is a decision that involves only a woman and her doctor, Cynthia knew of no other place to turn but to Planned Parenthood. So she made an appointment, drove herself to the clinic, and aborted her unborn child. Afterward, Cynthia was still successful at the office, but sometime later the nightlife ceased to interest her. Now, a single career woman with no husband and no children, Cynthia lies awake at night regretting her abortion.

Each of these women was torn and confused after finding out about her pregnancy and was either pressured or presented no other alternatives to aborting her baby. Often, women in these circumstances believe the lie that they are not carrying a child. "It's just a clump of tissue," the media assures them. In a matter of minutes, their abortion doctor takes the precious life growing within them. However, the memory of their baby lives on.

Stories like these echo the accounts of many of the million or so women in America per year who receive an abortion.[1] Though their backgrounds differ, their cries resound with the same grief, the same remorse, the same guilt and shame. Many hope deep down that someone will affirm what they know to be true in their hearts—that abortion is taking the life of another person. They long for someone to reassure them that there is another way forward. And if they did not feel this way before the abortion, they certainly do afterward.

While political campaigners and lobbyists tout the tagline that a woman has a right to choose to do with her body whatever she wants, arguments abound against such an appeal. Not only is abortion a death sentence for the unborn, it also leaves scars on the woman that last a lifetime—some physical, others emotional. For many women, it takes several years before they are able to tell their stories. Each of the women above has experienced redemption—indeed God forgives *all* things (1 John 1:9). But they openly admit that their pain has remained with them. It never goes away—not entirely. If only we could save the lives of these millions of unborn children. But an equally important mission is to rescue women in crisis, to help prevent the nights of tears and sleeplessness, and to spare them from the path of shame and guilt.

The Cultural War

If abortion is distressing to the lives of individual women, it has wreaked similar havoc on our contemporary public discourse.

Abortion has been and remains a hotly contested issue in American society, such that simply discussing the morality of abortion elicits passionate opinions on all sides of the social and political spectrum. This is due, on the one hand, to the very personal nature of the issue. Freedoms hang in the balance, and people will fight tooth and nail for the lives and liberties they seek to preserve. Still, abortion in America has become far more than a stand-alone issue. Our country is caught up in a contest between ideologies, in what some have called a *culture war*, and the abortion debate lies squarely at the center of the conflict.

Sociologist James Davison Hunter defines a *cultural conflict* as "political and social hostility rooted in different systems of moral understanding."[2] According to Hunter, "The end to which these hostilities tend is the domination of one cultural and moral ethos over all others," and the focus of the current conflict between Americans is over nothing less than the moral vision and values of our country. Battles erupt daily over hot topics—"abortion, child care, funding for the arts, affirmative action and quotas, gay rights, values in public education, or multiculturalism," to repeat Hunter's original list—but these are merely manifestations of a deeper ideological divide. The struggle is really a consequence of the incompatibility of our differing worldviews. "They are not merely attitudes that can change on a whim but basic commitments and beliefs that provide a source of identity, purpose, and togetherness for the people who live by them. It is for precisely this reason that political action rooted in these principles and ideals tends to be so passionate."[3]

The culture war has persisted in America for decades, with each side becoming gradually polarized and the rhetoric increasingly vicious. For moral conservatives, it is tempting to believe that if only more religious people would show up to vote that a sea change would occur in the policies and moral fabric of our country. Yet such a view probably attributes too much influence to the realm of politics. Besides that, lines can no longer be neatly drawn between religious and secular communities, as many who identify as religious, even Christian, support what are typically considered to be morally progressive positions and policies, including the right of women to choose to terminate unwanted pregnancies. According to a 2018 Gallup poll, 34 percent of those who identify as Protestant and 39 percent of those who identify as Catholic consider abortion to be "morally acceptable."[4]

These are sobering statistics. They reveal just how strongly the tide of progressive culture has pulled the church away from its biblical roots. We don't mean to sensationalize the situation in American Christianity, or to oversimplify all the relevant issues involving abortion and the other highly charged discussion points that frequent the media headlines. Of course, contemporary American politics are extremely complex, often requiring the informed Christian voter to weigh what are sometimes competing moral values as they advance their own priorities and at the same time "seek the welfare" of their fellow American image bearers (Jer. 29:7). More than that, the felt needs and suffering of women who face unplanned pregnancies are very real and should not be dismissed.

But with that said, how can Christians who believe that Jesus became human in order to redeem the human species relativize the worth of the most vulnerable of that species to the point where it is "morally acceptable" to terminate unborn lives? How should those who believe the biblical teaching on the sanctity of life answer the claims of their pro-choice peers? And how should believers in Jesus respond to the overwhelming political and societal pressure that progressive culture is mounting against evangelical Christianity?

A Call to Action

In a January 31, 2021, *Wall Street Journal* op-ed, Ryan T. Anderson, president of the Ethics & Public Policy Center, issued a simple call to action worth considering. Anderson advised cultural conservatives to respond directly yet intelligently to the pressures of their ideological opponents. "Americans need to figure out how to coexist peacefully on these issues," Anderson insisted. "But the answer isn't for our side to forfeit the fight about the truth by pleading only to be left alone. . . . We'll have the best shot at winning fights over abortion restrictions," Anderson argued, "when conservatives are willing to assert that their beliefs are true, not merely protected in law." According to Anderson, what is needed is for morally conservative thinkers to *engage* abortion defenders and other progressive ideologues, and to do so armed with cogent and rational argumentation—that which can't be easily dismissed on the basis of religion. "If we fail to fight back in the court of public opinion against the claim that our beliefs are 'bigoted,' we will ultimately lose even in courts of law, where the soundness of our beliefs is supposedly irrelevant. If basic truths of human nature are redefined as religious bigotry, they will be excised from society, in court and out."[5]

Anderson's call for peaceful, intellectual engagement on the matter of abortion is right on target for anyone who shares his convictions about the Bible's pro-life message and its teachings on how to engage one's ideological "other." "For the weapons of our warfare," announced the apostle Paul, "are not of the flesh but have divine power to destroy strongholds. We destroy arguments and every lofty opinion raised against the knowledge of God" (2 Cor. 10:4–5).

Yet the manner of our engagement is as equally important as the method. If we wish for American society ever again to respect—much less reflect—our cherished biblical values, then Christians must embody not only the boldness but the grace of our Lord Jesus Christ. We must engage, but do so peaceably (Rom. 12:18). We must speak the truth, but do so in love (Eph. 4:15). We must bear with the assaults of our critics, but do so with "compassionate hearts, kindness, humility, meekness, and patience" (Col. 3:12). This is all the more important when we step out from behind our mobile devices and social media pseudonyms and have real-life, enfleshed conversations with people we know and love. Indeed, if we ever wish to see our sister, daughter, niece, or neighbor choose life in the wake of an unplanned or unwanted pregnancy, we must arm ourselves with answers as well as empathy.

This book seeks to provide such answers, and to do so in a tone that takes seriously the anxiety and concerns of real women, and that models the way Christians ought to engage in public discourse.[6] With twenty essays authored by leading evangelical thinkers and activists, this volume offers Christians an accessible, charitable, yet well-argued resource for addressing the problem of abortion in our current cultural and political moment. By preparing the reader to answer pro-choice claims with confidence and compassion, we aim to equip Christians to defend prenatal life without compromising their gospel witness.

The Chapters at a Glance

Each of the chapters of this book is directed in response to one of seven common claims of abortion defenders.

Claim 1: "The courts have already settled the issue."

In chapter 1, "A More Excellent Way: Moral Decision-Making beyond Government Law," John Goodrich argues that true virtue and morality must operate within a system of ethics that considers morality beyond government legal prescription and proscription. Instead, people in general, but even more so followers of Jesus, must draw on the resources of *reason* to deduce natural law, and of *revelation* to discern biblical principles for decision-making, not least "the law of Christ" (Gal. 6:2)—the way of living in conformity to Jesus' self-giving and sacrifice motivated by love of others.

In "*Roe v. Wade*: Destined for the Dustbin," chapter 2, attorney Catherine Glenn Foster outlines various reasons why the landmark Supreme Court decision on abortion will inevitably be overturned. Foster reveals how widely criticized *Roe* is even within the legal community as well as how vulnerable it remains to reversal. This she demonstrates on the basis of the current composition of the Supreme Court, as well as the recent opinions the court justices have authored, which together point toward the eventual overturning of the ruling. Along the way, Foster shares her own disturbing story of forced abortion, the medical risks of abortion, and what it is going to take moving forward to make *Roe* a thing of the past.

Claim 2: "The fetus is not a person."

Chapter 3, "Made in God's Image: Personhood according to Scripture," examines those passages of Scripture that address prenatal life in order to answer the questions of whether the fetus is a person and thus whether the command "do not murder" applies to the unborn. Jeanette Hagen Pifer draws on a definition of personhood rooted in the biblical idea of being made in God's image and concludes that from God's perspective, there is a continuity of personal identity from inside to outside the womb—and thus the commandment not to murder absolutely applies to taking the life of the unborn.

In chapter 4, "More Than the Sum of Its Parts: Philosophical Reflections on Human Personhood," Scott Rae argues for a *substance view* of the human being that necessitates taking seriously the personhood and moral status of human embryos and fetuses. While various arguments have been advanced to suggest that the personhood of the human being should be assigned late in the developmental process, Rae demonstrates that each of these arguments relies only on arbitrary criteria for defining or detecting personhood.

"Knit Together in a Mother's Womb: The Biology of Prenatal Development." In chapter 5, Tara Sander Lee draws on the insights of recent scientific discovery to demonstrate that a new biological human being is created at the moment of conception. She walks the reader through the entire process of embryonic and fetal development, highlighting landmark moments of growth and effectively showing that a separate organism—indeed, a human person—is what is living and maturing within the pregnant woman.

From a legal standpoint, Joshua Craddock argues for the personhood of unborn humans on the basis of an originalist reading of the US Constitution in chapter 6, "Equal Protection for the Preborn: A Case for Prenatal Personhood according to the Fourteenth Amendment." Focusing on the Fourteenth Amendment, Craddock explains that the Amendment's protection of every "person" within the jurisdiction of the United States guarantees the same for the preborn, since "person" at the time of the Amendment's ratification was understood to encompass all members of the human species, born and unborn alike. His findings serve as the basis not only for overturning *Roe v. Wade* but also for the federal government's prohibiting of abortion even in those states that have adopted laws protecting abortion rights.

Claim 3: "My body, my choice."

In chapter 7, "Whose Body? The Illusion of Autonomy," Joy Riley disassembles the argument that the mother should have the right to abort simply because the fetus occupies *her* body, exposing the lie that abortion only involves the mother. Abortions implicate many others, including the distinct unborn person who is growing inside her, as well as the medical professionals who contribute to the taking of unborn life. Riley also shows that, from a Christian ethical perspective, there are other, more important factors to consider in abortion besides one's own "self-rule," namely that believers in Jesus are charged not to make decisions principally for their own good, but for the well-being of others.

In "Marvelously Revealed: The Symphony of a Woman's Body," chapter 8, Donna Harrison invites the reader to see afresh the beautiful intricacies of how a woman's body functions to prepare for and accommodate procreation. The female reproductive anatomy is nothing short of a gift from God. Indeed, a woman's body undergoes various awesome developments throughout pregnancy and over the course of her life. These changes not only bear God's fingerprints but demand that the woman's body be protected from the dangers of abortion, in order to ensure her medical well-being.

Claim 4: "I should not have to raise an unwanted child."

Bethany Bomberger responds to the lie propagandized for a century by Planned Parenthood that only "wanted" children should be brought into this world in chapter 9, "The Myth of the Unwanted Child: How Adoption Powerfully Dispels the Lie." Bomberger shows that in fact every child is wanted and has inherent value and purpose. Then after sharing her own family's involvement in adoption, Bomberger calls on all Christians to participate in the mission of adoption while encouraging women with unplanned pregnancies to consider entrusting their child to the care of an adoptive family.

In chapter 10, "Mom, Thank You for Choosing Life: The Perspective of an Abortion Survivor," Sarah Zagorski tells the inspiring yet heart-wrenching story of her own delivery—a failed abortion attempt that resulted in a standoff between her impoverished, immigrant mother and a notorious abortion physician over whether Sarah, a 26-week-old preemie, would live or die. She unpacks the complexities of her mother's story, which have led her to a place of increased empathy for women who consider abortion. Sarah calls Christians to love, not judge, these women in need, while encouraging these women to follow in her mother's steps by taking the courageous step of choosing life.

Claim 5: "My circumstances justify ending my pregnancy."

"Embracing Life's Bump: Experiencing God's Grace in Teenage Pregnancy." In chapter 11, Amy Ford invites the reader into her own account of teen pregnancy and of coming within moments of aborting her son. By God's grace, she was able to walk out of the abortion clinic and embrace the gift of motherhood. But her own experience lacked the support she now realizes is essential for teens who face unplanned pregnancies today. Teenage mothers require love and community, as well as various practical means of support to provide for themselves, to care for their child, and perhaps to finish school. Amy discusses all of this, as well as the possibility of adoption, in order to encourage and empower teen moms to choose life.

In chapter 12, "Hope Is Found in Hard Places: Pregnant during Financial Hardship," Christina Bennett tells the story of her mother, Andrea, whose providential encounter with a mysterious woman in the halls of the hospital empowered her to walk out of her abortion appointment and choose life—Christina's life. Andrea would go on to raise Christina and her brother as a single mother with very few resources. Yet Christina's childhood was full of love, and by perseverance and God's grace she has accomplished much. Christina uses her story and those of others as well as Scripture to encourage pregnant women with few resources to trust in God to provide for their needs, and never to find their identity in what they lack.

Chapter 13 is titled "But God Intended It for Good: Finding Purpose in Pregnancy from Rape." Paula Ilari, a woman who was gang raped but chose to carry and love her baby rather than abort, vividly retells the harrowing event that changed her forever. Yet despite the trauma of the experience, Paula has found peace and purpose in her son Caleb. This, she shares, is the outlook of most rape victims who decide to carry their babies. Thus, after narrating her assault and its aftermath, Paula offers a word of encouragement to mothers in similar circumstances. God, she assures us, is working to transform pain into purpose.

In chapter 14, "Fearfully and Wonderfully Made: Reimagining Pregnancy When the Baby Has Disabilities," Carlynn Fabarez shares the sobering account of being pregnant with her daughter, Stephanie, who was diagnosed during a routine ultrasound appointment with serious medical conditions. The doctor adamantly advised the couple to abort. But recognizing the sanctity of Stephanie's life regardless of her relative health, Carlynn and Mike courageously chose life and carried Stephanie for the length of the pregnancy, a decision that was made on the basis of scriptural truth. Seeking to provide strength for women facing pregnancies with similar medical complications, Carlynn shares with the reader ten biblically grounded reasons to choose life when fear and uncertainty assault one's heart.

"Are Abortions Ever Medically Necessary? A Life-Affirming Approach to Complex Pregnancies." In chapter 15, Kendra Kolb makes the case that abortion is never necessary to preserve the health or life of an expectant mother. While various medical conditions can seriously jeopardize a mother's well-being, what such pregnancies require is preterm delivery, not abortion. Not only are certain early delivery methods faster than abortion, but when performed past the point of viability, early deliveries often result in saving the life of not only the mother but the child, thanks to recent advances in medical technology. For this reason and others, Kolb argues that there is not a single maternal or fetal condition that necessitates the direct and intentional termination of preborn life in order to preserve the life of the mother.

Claim 6: "Abortions are helpful to women and society."

Victoria Robinson, author, speaker, and pro-life activist, shares from her own experience of having an abortion, as well as her experience counseling thousands of post-abortive women. In chapter 16, "The Truth about Post-Abortive Trauma: The Personal Account of a Survivor and Activist," Victoria outlines the devastating effects of abortion on both women and men, concluding that the consequences of abortion far surpass the challenge of an unplanned pregnancy.

In chapter 17, "An Expedient Tool: The Harmful Effects of Abortion on Society," Patrina Mosley demonstrates how abortion negatively impacts not only women and men, but broader society as well. In particular, Mosley exposes how Planned Parenthood is rooted in eugenics—the elite and powerful have promoted abortion in order to control the population of "those we don't want too many of." Often, abortion is touted as a tool for accomplishing good, but in reality it is nothing short of an expedient tool for producing evil.

Claim 7: "The pro-life movement doesn't care about social justice."

In chapter 18, "The Voices and Values of the New Pro-Life Generation," Charlotte Pence Bond, author, activist, and daughter of former Vice President Mike Pence, provides a window into the culture and convictions of young people today, arguing that the commitment of millennials and younger generations to upholding social justice has primed them to oppose the practice of elective abortion. Bond demonstrates on numerous counts why the pro-life movement is rightly understood to be a social justice movement, and then profiles several young leaders of the pro-life movement whose varied forms of activism have and will continue to inspire young people to advocate for the protection of the unborn.

Sandy Christiansen, in chapter 19, "The Hands and Feet of Jesus: How Pregnancy Centers Care for Women and Men," draws on her personal experience with and expert knowledge of pregnancy centers in order to dispel the myth that the pro-life movement cares only about unborn babies and not the others involved. Pregnancy centers stand at the frontlines of the pro-life movement providing a range of valuable services and a depth of care that brings healing to the whole person and the entire family, all free of charge. Local pregnancy centers are a safe place where expecting mothers and parents of newborns can turn for compassion, hope, and help in the name of Jesus.

"The Pro-Life Movement: A Last Line of Protection for Black Women and Their Babies." In chapter 20, Catherine Davis powerfully exposes how Planned Parenthood and its supporters have systematically targeted the Black community from the very inception of the abortion industry in America. After surveying the early history of this organization's attempts to disguise this targeting, Davis examines how Planned Parenthood has rebranded itself in recent years in order to deflect negative publicity, while strategically targeting the pro-life movement and pregnancy resource centers in order to suppress the pro-life message.

Our Hope

Whether the book is read cover to cover, or only selectively in order to grow in one's understanding of specific issues, we hope this resource will equip the reader with cogent, rational argumentation that is at the same time grace-filled and Christ-honoring. It is our desire to prepare readers to engage in the abortion debate with answers and empathy, reason and understanding, confidence and compassion. In doing so, we hope that more women, like Elizabeth, Lydia, and Cynthia, will find the help they need before making the life-altering decision to abort their babies.

CLAIM 1

The Courts Have Already Settled the Issue

1

A More Excellent Way: Moral Decision-Making beyond Government Law

—John K. Goodrich—

Like many people, I love a good courtroom drama. Whether fictional and comedic, like *My Cousin Vinny*, or based on historical events, like *Erin Brockovich*, I become easily engrossed in the performance of on-screen lawyers—their careful investigative work, their intense deposing of star witnesses, and most of all their shrewd dissection of legal arguments as they attempt to win the case.

Without question, my favorite trial movie of all time is *A Few Good Men*. In the film, Tom Cruise plays Lt. Daniel Kaffee, a recent Harvard Law School alum and talented JAG officer who is notorious for taking more interest in sporting events than in defending his clients. One of the more enjoyable legal segments of the film doesn't even take place in a courtroom. In the scene where we first meet Kaffee, the lieutenant is approached during softball practice by prosecutor Lt. David Spradling, who interrupts the team's fielding drills to plea bargain a pending drug charge against one of Kaffee's clients. Midway through the exchange, Spradling presents the charge and begins the negotiation. Kaffee immediately rejects the offer, because as it turns out, his client hadn't actually been caught with an illegal substance. Instead, the defendant had mistakenly bought what amounted to ten dollars' worth of oregano. "Yeah, well, your client thought it was marijuana," Spradling asserted. "My client's a moron," Kaffee replied. "That's not against the law."[1]

This interaction between the two lieutenants comedically illustrates the manner in which many people in our society, even some self-avowed Christians, seek to justify their decision-making. They assume that as long as they have not broken the law, they can rest assured that they are morally upright people. Some even believe an action is wrong only when a lawbreaker gets caught—though that is a different ethical problem altogether.

But are legal statutes alone capable of providing everything we need for consistently making moral decisions? Doesn't discerning right from wrong, moral from immoral, require us to consider matters beyond what the law forbids? More to the point, does the Supreme Court's ruling on *Roe v. Wade* really establish that abortion is a *morally* legitimate choice?

The truth is there are too many people in our society who make significant, life-altering decisions simply on the basis of the legality of their options. And the same is true with respect to abortion, as Rebecca Todd Peters acknowledges—in fact, applauds—in her recent "progressive Christian" defense of the pro-choice position. "For many women," Peter maintains, "abortion is *not* a moral dilemma. It is not a dilemma, because they do not want to be pregnant (for any number of reasons), *the procedure is legal in this country,* and we have the medical knowledge of how to safely terminate their pregnancy.

These women feel no moral obligation to carry every pregnancy to term. They are simply sexually active women who have gotten pregnant."[2]

To be fair, Peters is not necessarily speaking for herself, but is reporting, although approvingly, what she perceives to be true of other women. Nevertheless, her declaration that the mere legalization of abortion (together with the relative safety of the procedure and a person's desire to obtain one) provides the moral ground needed to terminate a pregnancy is a striking admission. And it ultimately raises the question about how we, as morally culpable human beings, ought to determine right from wrong.

In this essay we will explain why moral decision-making requires more than taking our moral cues from local or federal legislation—that is, more than what we will call *legal positivism*.[3] This is especially true for those of us who claim to be followers of Jesus Christ. First, we will discuss the benefits of societal laws before exposing their inability alone to provide sufficient moral guidance. We will then explore how God expects Christians to engage in moral reasoning by introducing the two primary sources available to us for making moral judgments. Finally, we will examine how those two sources for discerning morality should factor into our evaluation about whether abortion is ethically permissible.

Government Law

The Bible consistently affirms the importance of establishing national laws and appointing government leaders in order to execute justice in keeping with those laws. David acclaims that the law God gave to Israel is perfect and revives the soul (Ps. 19:7). In fact, it is the righteousness of this law that was supposed to signal Israel's greatness before all its neighbors (Deut. 4:5–8). Thus, God promised that if the Israelites obeyed His commandments, they would indeed prosper (Deut. 30:15–16), and that if Israel's king himself were to obey the law, the length of his reign would be great (Deut. 17:18–20).

The Bible also has much to say about the importance of governing authorities. Although such leaders are rebuked in Scripture from time to time (1 Cor. 2:6–8), the Bible repeatedly instructs its readers to recognize that God Himself has appointed rulers to their particular positions of leadership. God's people should therefore submit themselves to the governing authorities, so long as such obedience does not result in compromising God's other moral standards—"We must obey God rather than men" (Acts 5:29). Thus, in the Old Testament, God repeatedly reminds Israel's exiles that, even when they are under the rule of a foreign king, God remains sovereign still, for "the Most High rules the kingdom of men and gives it to whom he will" (Dan. 4:17, 25, 32). It is for this reason that Paul instructs believers living in the heart of the Roman empire, "Let every person be subject to the governing authorities. For there is no authority except from God, and those that exist have been instituted by God. Therefore whoever resists the authorities resists what God has appointed" (Rom. 13:1–2).

Despite the many public benefits that national laws and leaders provide, the Bible is also clear that the rulers and judges of this world should not be trusted uncritically (1 Cor. 6:1–6). Governments have been appointed to reward good and to curb evil (Rom. 13:3–4), but when someone relies exclusively or even primarily on legal systems, politicians, or judicial bodies to discern right from wrong, they will inevitably find themselves incapable of living a consistently moral life. As Christian ethicist Scott Rae so clearly explains, "the law is the *moral minimum*. Obeying the law is the beginning of our moral obligations, not the end."[4] What Rae is suggesting is that sometimes law and ethics do not agree. In fact, decisions are routinely required of us as human beings that either contradict or extend beyond the purview of the law. Ethicist Deni Elliott clarifies this point when she observes, "Legal and ethical guidelines are not the same. A proposed action may be 1) both legal and ethical, 2) legal but not ethical, 3) ethical but not legal, or 4) neither legal nor ethical."[5] When law and ethics agree, decision-making is typically easy. Unfortunately, this is not always the case. "Most of the pressing demands of morality," Rae maintains, "are in those spaces where the law is not definitive, where the law is silent, or where the law allows one to do something unethical."[6] And for that reason, it is important to distinguish what is *legal* from what is *ethical*, what we *can* do versus what we *should* do, and then commit to doing what is right.

A couple of examples of this discrepancy will help to illustrate the point. It is clear to the vast majority of people today, for instance, that racial discrimination is immoral. Yet racial segregation was legal in the United States as recently as 1964. Does that mean it was morally acceptable during or before the Jim Crow era of America's history for an individual to discriminate against another person on the basis of race? No, absolutely not. Regardless of what the law permitted, it was the moral responsibility of all people then—just as it is now and at all times—to treat one another with dignity and respect, despite racial or ethnic differences.

The same discrepancy is apparent in the case of marital infidelity. Despite the attraction of younger generations to lifestyles involving open relationships and polyamory, the vast majority of people agree that committed couples should be monogamous.[7] In Western societies, however, no criminal statutes exist to prevent or discourage someone from acting unfaithfully to their marriage partner. Does this suggest it is morally acceptable for a person to cheat on their spouse? No, not at all. Even without laws that would enforce marital fidelity, it is the moral responsibility of all people at all times to be faithful to their spouse for as long as they remain married.

Additional examples could easily be provided (e.g., lying, murder, profanity), but the validity of the above two normative moral principles should be immediately clear to most people, even if no laws exist to enforce them. Is the same true of abortion? Is intentionally ending the life of a preborn baby morally problematic even though abortion is legal in most contemporary Western societies? And how can we know? In our final two sections we will explore the two primary sources of moral authority that people should consider as they seek to make ethical decisions that extend beyond the reach of government law.

Natural Law

In place of *legal positivism* (the determination of right and wrong based simply on what the law permits), the better way for Christians, and all people, to decipher how they should and should not conduct their lives is by drawing upon the natural and supernatural sources from which moral standards are knowable in our world. In other words, we need to use both *reason* and *revelation*. In this section we will explore the former, and in the next section we will examine the latter.

When we seek to discern right and wrong by observing the natural order of the world, we are drawing upon "natural law." Rae defines natural law as the "general, objective, and widely shared moral values that are not specifically tied to the special revelation of

Scripture"—values like justice, truth, human dignity, and the preservation of life.[8] "These values," Rae continues, "are a consensus that comes out of the observations and conclusions of humankind over the centuries. In the same way that God has revealed truth about the sciences in creation and revealed truth in the observations of humankind in the social sciences, natural law refers to God's revelation of morality from all sources outside of Scripture. In this sense, natural law is general revelation applied to moral values."[9] Of course, there will be people in every society and in every time period who will disagree with this or that moral norm. But the fact that there exists general agreement on numerous ethical issues across most people groups helps to establish the validity of natural law.

What, then, does natural law teach us about the morality of abortion? In brief, natural law suggests that abortion is *immoral*. Obviously, this is not universally recognized today, nor has it been throughout history, so this moral point cannot be established simply by appealing to historical consensus (the same, of course, is true of slavery and sex trafficking).[10] Nevertheless, it is important to note that a slight majority of Americans agrees that abortion is immoral, as recent Gallup polls demonstrate.[11] Even though the statistical evidence is not overwhelming, we can explain the lack of consensus at least in part by appealing to the failure of many people to recognize the humanity and personhood of the unborn. In other words, once basic science is allowed to enter the discussion, popular arguments in favor of abortion often unravel. And thanks to the scientific advances of the last century, compelling arguments for the immorality of abortion are gaining wider acceptance.

The natural law argument against the morality of abortion is proven by demonstrating three simple premises. *First,* from the moment of conception (fertilization), an unborn entity is a full-fledged member of the human community. *Second,* it is morally wrong to kill any member of the human community. *Third,* every successful abortion kills a full-fledged member of the human community. *Therefore,* every successful abortion is morally wrong.[12]

The second and third of these premises hardly require defending, since they are already widely accepted. After all, regarding premise two, most people and basically all civilized societies recognize that killing human beings is immoral. This is because all humans have a fundamental right to life, and killing someone results in the permanent, irreversible denial of that right.[13] Exceptions to this rule have been observed—for instance, in circumstances of just war, self-defense, and capital punishment—though these examples remain hotly contested and do not apply to the case of abortion. Furthermore, some have defended abortion by appealing to how an unborn child's right to life conflicts with the mother's right to liberty—that is, her right to control her own body. However, as Robert Spitzer explains, "Objective necessity requires that the child's right to life supersede the mother's right to liberty, because life is the necessary condition for the possibility of liberty."[14]

Moreover, regarding premise three, all people considering an abortion recognize that a successful procedure terminates whatever unborn entity is in their womb, whether they consider it to be a person or an appendage. As Carol Sanger asserts, "Women—even young women—understand very well what an abortion is. They understand that abortion ends pregnancy and that if they have an abortion, they will not have a baby: that is its very point."[15]

The real debate, therefore, centers on the validity of the first premise—the humanity and personhood of the unborn. Chapters 4, 5, and 6 of this volume provide comprehensive defenses of fetal personhood from natural law perspectives, making the case through appeal to philosophy, biology, and law. For now, I will present only a brief argument for the humanity of the unborn by demonstrating that the overwhelming consensus among expert scientists is that human life begins at conception (fertilization).

Recent scientific literature has established that life, and thus humanness, begins at fertilization. Embryologist Brian Dale makes this link in his aptly titled book *Fertilization: The Beginning of Life*, in which he writes that fertilization is the "fascinating process where two highly specialized cells interact to form a *new life*."[16] The same point is made by Samuel Webster and Rhiannon de Wreede in their textbook *Embryology at a Glance*: "Animals begin life as a single cell. That cell must produce new cells and form increasingly complex structures in an organised and controlled manner to reliably and successfully build a new organism. . . . Embryology is the branch of biology that studies the early formation and development of these organisms. Embryology begins with fertilisation."[17] Ronan O'Rahilly and Fabiola Müller agree in their book *Human Embryology and Teratology*: "It needs to be emphasized that life is continuous, as is also human life, so that the question 'When does (human) life begin?' is meaningless in terms of ontogeny [i.e., the development of an organism]. Although life is a continuous process, fertilization . . . is a critical landmark because, under ordinary circumstances, *a new genetically distinct human organism is formed* when the chromosomes of the male and female pronuclei blend in oocyte [i.e., in the egg]."[18]

If these handpicked excerpts were not enough,[19] a recent University of Chicago doctoral dissertation shows this to be nothing less than the consensus opinion of the academic community. Through a survey that received responses from over 5,500 biologists from more than 1,000 leading universities around the globe, Steven Andrew Jacobs has demonstrated that an overwhelming percentage of life science professionals agree that life begins at fertilization. According to Jacobs, each of the scientists he surveyed was asked to affirm or reject five statements that in various ways endorse fertilization as the moment when life commences. Of the 5,557 respondents, "only 240 participants did not affirm at least one of the statements (4%)," "86% affirmed at least half of the items they assessed, and 64% affirmed each item they assessed. Thus, regardless of the phrasing of the question," Jacobs summarizes, "a majority of biologists [as high as 96%] affirm the underlying biological view that a human's life begins at fertilization."[20] "These data," he concludes, "would then not only suggest that fetuses are biological humans but that fetuses are humans because they are developing in the human life cycle."[21] That being the case, the first premise of the natural law argument for the immorality of abortion is secure.

Admittedly, there are abortion defenders who grant that embryos and fetuses are humans because they have the right genetic material. However, these same people deny that unborn humans are persons and have the right to life. This is because, according to their understanding, a human becomes a person sometime after fertilization, whether late in pregnancy or even after birth. Answering this claim requires a much lengthier discussion than we have space for here. I will leave it to chapters 4 to 6 to respond to these arguments from a natural law perspective, and to chapter 3 from a biblical perspective. For now, I will simply say that it is entirely arbitrary to assign the beginning of personhood to a moment or developmental phase following conception.[22] Attempts to do so eventually lead to problems in a variety of other cases involving the sanctity of life. Thus, it is best to assign personhood to any and all human beings, regardless of age or functional ability. Provided, then, the accuracy of the first, second, and third premises of the argument made above, the natural law argument against the morality of abortion is sound.

The Law of Christ

We have just seen that natural law theorists spend their time showing how the universal availability of reason makes all humanity responsible for keeping rationally discernable moral truths. Theologians, on the other hand, maintain that moral absolutes have also been revealed through inspired Scripture. Here we will survey some of the principles derived from the Bible that inform how we should make moral decisions in general, and how we should respond to the abortion epidemic in particular.

In the Old Testament, God prescribes the Law of Moses as the behavioral standard His people were to live by as they sought to maintain a relationship with Him. The New Testament, however, is quick to point out that obedience to the Mosaic Law is neither sufficiently possible nor ultimately necessary for those who are believers in Jesus. Indeed, Paul announces that "we are released from the law, having died to that which held us captive, so that we serve in the new way of the Spirit and not in the old way of the written code" (Rom. 7:6).

Now, while followers of Jesus are not obligated to keep the commandments of Moses in order to maintain a relationship with God, their lives should reflect the core principles of the divine law as they seek to love God with their entire selves, and to love others as themselves (Matt. 22:36–40; citing Deut. 6:5; Lev. 19:18). As Paul charges the believers in Galatia, "you were called to freedom [from the law], brothers. Only do not use your freedom as an opportunity for the flesh, but through love serve one another. For the whole law is fulfilled in one word: 'You shall love your neighbor as yourself'" (Gal. 5:13–14; citing Lev. 19:18). The legal statutes that Paul insists Christians have been freed from are the 613 commandments belonging to the Law of Moses—not law codes established by contemporary political and legislative bodies. In place of the Mosaic Law, Christians are to live in the Spirit and thereby pursue a lifestyle characterized by a particular virtue—namely, *love of others*. By living in the Spirit and loving others, Christians will, counterintuitively, fulfill the law.

Paul has a clever label for this principled mode of living—"the law of Christ." Paul instructs the Galatians, "Bear one another's burdens, and so fulfill the law of Christ" (Gal. 6:2). Biblical scholar Thomas Schreiner explains, "The 'law of Christ' is equivalent to the law of love ([Gal.] 5:13–14), so that when believers carry the burdens of others, they behave as Christ did and fulfill his law. In this sense Christ's life and death also become the paradigm, exemplification, and explanation of love."[23] Such burden carrying takes many forms in the modern church, though its defining feature is self-sacrifice for the benefit of others. For just as Jesus gave of Himself for all people, so believers should imitate Jesus' generosity by giving of themselves for the well-being of their fellow humans; believers are instructed to "do nothing from selfish ambition or conceit, but in humility count others more significant than yourselves. Let each of you look not only to his own interests, but also to the interests of others" (Phil. 2:3–4). Applying this ethic is not the result of the believer's own willpower alone. Christians are recipients of the Holy Spirit and thereby divinely transformed into the likeness of Christ as they are enabled to obey God and love people. It is for this reason that Paul can say that "the fruit of the Spirit is love" (Gal. 5:22).

There are additional moral qualities believers ought to exhibit as a result of the Holy Spirit's work in their lives, but this brief overview is sufficient to demonstrate that *Christian ethics* is ultimately a form of *virtue ethics*. Rather than being defined by a laundry list of "dos and don'ts" (though there are certainly many black-and-white moral norms prescribed by the biblical authors), the Christian teaching on morality principally involves God's people becoming like Jesus Christ, by internalizing His character traits and living them out in the circumstances and relationships of everyday life.

Let's elaborate further on how to make virtuous decisions by focusing our attention on Romans 12. In this passage, Paul calls Christians to "be transformed by the renewal of [their] mind," so they might make good moral choices—that is, so they can "discern what is the will of God, what is good and acceptable and perfect" (Rom. 12:2). At least part of what it means to have one's mind renewed and to discern God's will is addressed in the remainder of the passage, as Paul progresses from topics like the "mind" and discernment (12:2) to modest thinking and "sober judgment" (12:3). In other words, Christian decision-making fundamentally involves *humility*. The believer must adopt a humble estimation of one's own self-importance—committing "not to think of himself more highly than he ought to think, but to think with sober judgment" (12:3). Next, Christian decision making requires *integrity*. The believer must determine to do what is right and to resist doing what is wrong regardless of the circumstances—committing to "abhor what is evil" and "hold fast to what is good" (12:9). Finally, Christian decision-making demands *generosity*. The believer must give oneself for others—finding concrete ways to "love one another with brotherly affection" and to "outdo one another in showing honor" (12:10). These principles, Paul assures us, will guide us faithfully as we seek to live out God's mercies in our decision-making as new creatures in Christ.

The practical implications of these biblical principles for the morality of abortion should be clear. Here I will highlight two. *First, Christian men and women should value the lives of the unborn.* As people called to "love your neighbor" and to care for "the least of these" (Luke 10:25–37; Matt. 25:40), Christians must recognize that there is no one on earth who is as much a neighbor to a pregnant woman as her unborn child, and no one who is more vulnerable and in greater dependence on another person as a child in utero. Thus, the love of Christ compels His followers to value unborn lives. This mandate to love does not only apply to the mother and father of an unborn child; it also applies to the baby's entire family and their whole community. And of course, this love should not evaporate once the baby arrives. Often, that is when the needs of the child and of the parents become greater. But this love should be present even during pregnancy.

Second, Christian men and women should go to great lengths to ensure the survival and safe delivery of unborn children. There are many reasons why women consider abortion, and even why they might believe abortion to be a morally acceptable decision. Pro-choice author Rebecca Todd Peters asserts, "In circumstances where pregnancy or parenting a child, or an additional child, represents undue physical, financial, or psychological hardship, the possibility of an abortion represents a *moral good* that secures a woman's well-being and often the well-being of her existing family."[24] But is this true? How is extinguishing innocent life good for anybody? And what about the well-being of the *baby*? Christians must love others in such a way that they put the good and well-being of vulnerable unborn children above their own convenience, preferences, and supposed well-being. During pregnancy, no one can replace the mother in the care of her unborn child. No one else can consume the right foods, breathe the right air, protect the baby from alcohol and narcotics, or protect the baby from those who believe preborn life is dispensable. As people who value and prioritize the lives of the unborn, Christians must therefore be willing to care for their own children and to see their pregnancies through to birth.

Conclusion

Morality and legality are not the same thing. Considering what the law sanctions and prohibits is *significant* to our moral decision making, but it is never *sufficient* for deciding right from wrong. The morally conscious person must also consider the moral norms revealed through both natural law and the Bible. Reason (natural law) shows us that human life begins at conception, and thus even the earliest stages of human development must be protected. Moreover, because revelation (the Bible) calls God's people to live generously and sacrificially, Christians must advocate for the protection of unborn children and go to great lengths to help the mothers of unplanned pregnancies, even at great expense to themselves. Followers of Jesus are called to consider not merely what the *government permits*, but what *God expects*. And God expects those devoted to Him to make moral decisions based on the standards of morality revealed in Scripture, modelled by Jesus, and encoded into the transformed hearts of God's Spirit-indwelt followers. This virtue-based mode of decision-making is what Paul calls "a more excellent way" (1 Cor. 12:31) and it should lead all Christians, indeed all people, to *choose life*.

2

Roe v. Wade: Destined for the Dustbin

—Catherine Glenn Foster—

In fall 2019, when the leaves were just starting to turn and months before the coronavirus pandemic hit America, the National Constitution Center invited me to Philadelphia to debate two abortion-rights advocates, Kathryn (Kitty) Kolbert and Mary Ziegler. Kolbert is the ACLU attorney who "saved" *Roe v. Wade* in 1992 when she stood before the US Supreme Court and harangued the Justices that they "could not go back" on "abortion rights." Ziegler, a law professor at Florida State University, has written a number of books and articles about abortion, and in 2020 put her name on a brief filed in the Supreme Court asking the Court to continue following *Roe v. Wade* and to uphold the constitutional right to abortion it had fashioned back in 1973.

To my surprise, in a televised forum before a studio audience that night, Kolbert and Ziegler both declared that "this Court will overturn *Roe v. Wade*." While I was glad to hear such a concession from these two high-profile abortion-rights advocates, I sensed that it was really intended to inspire abortion activists to action, and I took it with a grain of salt. I also knew that the road won't be easy. Numerous hurdles—legal, electoral, and political—stand in the way of overturning *Roe v. Wade*. And yet I'm convinced that it will happen, sooner or later.

Still Unsettled

I suppose it is difficult for many Americans to understand why the political and legal battle against *Roe v. Wade* has gone on for so long. Why isn't *Roe v. Wade* settled after forty-seven years, eleven presidential elections, and an entire turnover in the membership of the US Supreme Court?

First and foremost, the *Roe* decision is *fatally flawed*. It was bad constitutional law then, and it is bad constitutional law now. Not only that, the process within the Supreme Court that produced *Roe* was arbitrary and capricious, without a factual record on abortion or its risks and implications, which violated normal constitutional standards and procedures. All this has been widely conceded over the decades, even by those who like the result; a host of progressive legal professionals have acknowledged *Roe*'s fallacious reasoning:

As Justice Ruth Bader Ginsburg said in 1985: "*Roe,* I believe, would have been more acceptable as a judicial decision if it had not gone beyond a ruling on the extreme statute before the Court. . . . Heavy-handed judicial intervention was difficult to justify and appears to have provoked, not resolved, conflict."[1]

Or legal scholar John Hart Ely in 1973: "[*Roe*] is *not* constitutional law and gives almost no sense of an obligation to try to be. . . . What is frightening about *Roe* is that this super-protected right is not inferable from the language of the Constitution, the framers' thinking respecting the specific problem in issue, any general value derivable from the provisions they included, or the nation's governmental structure. . . . At times the inferences the Court has drawn from the values the Constitution marks for special protection have been controversial, even shaky, but never before has its sense of an obligation to draw one been so obviously lacking."[2]

Or Harvard Law Professor Laurence Tribe in 1973: "One of the most curious things about *Roe* is that, behind its own verbal smokescreen, the substantive judgment on which it rests is nowhere to be found."[3]

Or Harvard Law Professor Mark Tushnet in 1983: "It seems to be generally agreed that, as a matter of simple craft, Justice Blackmun's opinion for the Court was dreadful."[4]

Or University of Pennsylvania Law School Professor Kermit Roosevelt in 2003: "It is time to admit in public that, as an example of the practice of constitutional opinion writing, *Roe* is a serious disappointment. . . . As constitutional argument, *Roe* is barely coherent. The court pulled its fundamental right to choose more or less from the constitutional ether."[5]

Or Jeffrey Rosen (later president of the National Constitution Center) in 2003: "[*Roe*'s] overturning would be the best thing that could happen to the federal judiciary, the pro-choice movement, and the moderate majority of the American people. . . . Thirty years after *Roe,* the finest constitutional minds in the country still have not been able to produce a constitutional justification for striking down restrictions on early-term abortions that is substantially more convincing than Justice Harry Blackmun's famously artless opinion itself."[6]

The above concerns over *Roe v. Wade* are just the tip of the iceberg when it comes to the immense criticism the precedent has suffered over the years, coming from every part of the political spectrum and each pointing toward the eventual abandonment of the decision.

The decision overturned centuries of Anglo-American legal heritage protecting prenatal children to the greatest extent possible. As Dr. John Keown, the Rose F. Kennedy Professor of Christian Ethics at the Kennedy Institute of Ethics at Georgetown University, has observed: "*Roe* was a radical break with the law's historical protection of the unborn child and thereby with its adherence to the principle of the inviolability of human life."[7] Those protections were prevalent in the common law, which originated in England and traveled with her colonists to the early United States. In William Blackstone's comprehensive analysis of the English common law, he wrote on the subject that "if a woman is quick with child, and by a potion or otherwise, killeth it in her womb . . . this, though not murder, was by the ancient law homicide or manslaughter."[8] *Roe,* then, was a significant divergence from the common law history of America and the Western world at large.

Roe is extreme by international standards. Because of *Roe,* the United States is one of only five nations (along with the motley crew of Canada, China, North Korea, and Vietnam) that allows abortion for any reason after fetal viability, and one of only seven nations that allows abortion for any reason after 20 weeks of pregnancy.

Abortion disregards the science of embryology and fetal development. Ultrasound came on the commercial medical market in the United States just a few years after the *Roe* decision and blindsided the Justices. Ultrasound has provided a relevant and nearly universal window to the womb, permanently changed public understanding of human development, and helped spur growing state legal protections for children in utero.

The majority of the medical profession rejects abortion. Only a small percentage of doctors—approximately 14 percent—will perform abortions in the United States. Except for medical organization elites, like the leaders of the American Medical Association (AMA) and the American College of Obstetricians & Gynecologists (ACOG), the American medical profession has largely abandoned elective abortion.

The Supreme Court in *Roe* assumed an unprecedented, self-appointed role as the "national abortion control board." As a series of Justices have charged, the Court in *Roe* assumed the role of "the Nation's '*ex officio* medical board with powers to approve or disapprove medical and operative practices and standards throughout the United States.'"[9] But the Court doesn't have the tools to competently fill that role. The 2020 edition of *Unsafe*, Americans United for Life's national survey of abortion businesses and doctors, documents that "more than 300 abortion facilities in 39 states were cited for more than 2,400 health and safety deficiencies between 2008 and 2020."[10]

When the broad scope of *Roe* is understood, the ruling is supported by only a small minority of Americans. Unfortunately, that minority support is artificially inflated by the media and a number of billionaires and billion-dollar foundations. But perhaps most importantly, the majority of Americans and a broad, grassroots movement across the nation will not let *Roe* rest. The pro-life movement has worked for decades now to protect women and children from the harms of abortion, but in pursuit of consistency, has likewise spurred many states to move forward with legal protections for children in the womb even outside the context of abortion.

Abortion Hurts Women

The sweeping right to elective abortion that *Roe* decreed—for any reason, at any stage of pregnancy, in all fifty states—has harmed women's health and relationships. That reality has been obscured by the lack of any reliable national system of abortion data collection—which is a grave problem on its own for reporting and analysis—and by Planned Parenthood's marketing of abortion as "basic healthcare" for women.

Roe changed American culture. By legalizing a broad right, *Roe* leveraged the pressure of uncommitted men and subjected women to enormous pressure from men who don't want a baby and can escape financial responsibility if the baby never reaches birth. *Roe* isolated the woman in her decision-making under the guise of "privacy." The worst impact has fallen on poor women who get pregnant, as *Roe*'s proclamation of a "constitutional right" makes it seem unreasonable for any poor woman to refuse an abortion, especially if it is publicly funded.

Roe also changed the workplace for women. Within a few years, it was obvious to women and lawmakers that the right to abortion empowered employers to force women to choose between their *job* or their *pregnancy*. Congress had to pass the federal Pregnancy Discrimination Act in 1976 to protect pregnant women in the workplace; many states followed.

Furthermore, *Roe* changed the sexual marketplace in America. In a 2011 review, law professor Helen Alvaré explained that "legalized abortion has helped create and perpetuate a 'mating market' for women which is deeply at odds not only with their objective good, but also with their preferences."[11] Economists and sociologists have published studies that "provide a powerful warrant for laws and policies both to reduce abortion's availability in order to curb its 'insurance effect' in connection with uncommitted sexual encounters, and to reduce women's participation in nonmarital sexual relations, which have become the required 'currency' for women's participation in this mating market."[12]

Roe enabled sex-selection abortion in the United States and helped to encourage it around the globe. Numbers vary, but some researchers have documented the tragedy of 160,000,000 missing girls due to sex selection abortions worldwide.[13]

Roe struck down every abortion law in all fifty states, creating a legal vacuum in the regulation of abortion and the protection of women and children. The Court couldn't fill that vacuum, but rather put the burden on the states to do so—or not. Many states have tried to fill that vacuum. Some states have done very little.

Through *Roe,* the Supreme Court, directly or through the lower federal courts, has obstructed the enforcement of many health and safety laws passed by the states. For example, in June 2020 in the *June Medical Services v. Russo* case the Court struck down a protective Louisiana health and safety law. Emergency transfer laws, like the one *June Medical* considered, ensure that women who seek an abortion can access timely and lifesaving emergency medical care in the event of an incident during the abortion procedure, such as a perforated uterus. The rule requiring doctors who perform abortions to have admitting privileges at a nearby hospital was not unusual; in fact, all other outpatient surgeons in Louisiana are required to abide by that rule. But with the Supreme Court eliminating emergency transfer laws, abortion facilities are empowered to provide women with subpar care that endangers their patients' lives with no repercussions.

Abortion harms women and their relationships. Abortion does

not heal or restore male-female relationships; more often, it ends relationships. All too many women are coerced into abortion by their partners, parents, institutions, or peers. Most egregiously, for the pregnant victims of human trafficking, abortion is a cheap solution. And while some women "shout their abortion," many thousands of women have testified that abortion has injured them physically, psychologically, and emotionally.

I am one of them; I know the tragedy of abortion firsthand.

When I was nineteen years old, I walked through the doors of an abortion facility. I had never really thought much about abortion until it confronted me personally. I had heard the terms *pro-life, pro-choice* a couple of times, but that word *abortion* was almost unspoken. I didn't know what it was until, as a sophomore at a small college in Georgia, just back from Christmas break, I found myself unexpectedly pregnant. I had no idea where to turn.

I didn't know there was a pro-life movement, didn't know what help was out there. I had no idea where to go for nonjudgmental care. I was thinking, what do I do? Where do I go? I felt completely helpless. That night, like so many girls, I turned to the internet. What I found online was abortion facilities; they were the first things that popped up. I made an appointment for that Saturday. I didn't know for sure what I would do, but I knew that if I did end up getting an abortion, it would have to be fast, because I was already bonding with my child.

I remember that week vividly. I was wearing my boyfriend's oversized sweatshirt, and actually talking out loud with my baby as I walked around campus. I named her.

But on Saturday I opened the doors of that abortion business. And from the moment I walked in, nothing felt right. Nothing restored my choice, my autonomy, my sense of empowerment. It was just stripped from me over and again by everything that happened behind those closed doors. I asked questions, but got no answers. I asked to see the ultrasound, but they refused. And after I lay down on the table, I changed my mind. Something just clicked for me in that moment. I knew I was carrying a human being, a life. I knew that the abortion was wrong.

I tried to get up; I said, "Let me go. You can keep the money, but this is just wrong for me." I felt it in my heart and in my soul, that I couldn't go through with it. They shouted for backup. And in the end, I had a worker holding each arm, a worker holding each leg, and they held me down and forcibly aborted my baby. I could feel this indescribable pain. I knew exactly what was happening; it felt like a soul being ripped out of me. I was crying. I was screaming. They tried to cover me up so I would be quiet. And then, as quickly as it began, it was over.

I was the last patient to leave the clinic alive that day. I did not want to leave; I knew it would be the last time I would be with my baby. My boyfriend drove me back to college, about an hour and a half away. And I remember lying in bed for days, not wanting to move, not knowing how to go on. It was so incredibly traumatic. But that is the story of abortion across America. I have met so many women with similar stories. Abortion hurts women, and it hurt me.

The Risks of Abortion

The Supreme Court, disregarding the impact of abortion on women and society, broadly legalized the procedure as a "constitutional right." This means that abortion is treated differently from other medical procedures in the United States and is more exempt from legal regulation than other medical procedures.

Ninety-eight percent of the time, abortion is an *elective* procedure, not advised or done to treat a medical condition, not "medically indicated" but performed only for *social* reasons. It does not fix a health problem. Artificially ending a healthy pregnancy is not necessary for and does not contribute to women's health. There is no medical condition such that a doctor would advise alternative medical treatments to the abortion, and there is no comparison between abortion and medical procedures that treat a medical condition.

Consequently, women don't get comprehensive and detailed information about the short-term or long-term risks of abortion because the medical risks are considered irrelevant to the social desire for the termination of the pregnancy. The elective nature of abortion skews the informed consent process. A doctor has no need to discuss the pros and cons of medical alternatives. The short-term and long-term risks are largely beside the point of the social decision. One of the great tragedies of *Roe*, then, is that many women don't get fully informed consent and don't get a full picture of the short-term and long-term risks. If a state has passed no law requiring informed consent for abortion, women are dependent on what the abortion facility tells her about abortion—its nature, alternatives, and risks.

And in the United States, there is the additional problem that abortionists separate themselves from general OB-GYN practice, and abortion facilities seek self-regulation by operating in standalone surgi-centers. Since abortions aren't performed by a woman's regular OB-GYN, the abortion is rarely made part of her general medical records.

There is better data on abortion from outside the United States because many other countries, like Denmark and Finland, track every abortion through a national registry. That contributes to a woman's long-term health monitoring and counseling, provides a reliable body of evidence for research and data, and improves women's ability to give real informed consent.

Based in large part on the more reliable international data, the medical evidence of the impact of abortion on women has grown over the past three decades. Some have dismissed the evidence. Some medical organizations, like the American College of Obstetricians & Gynecologists (ACOG), even actively work with abortion advocates and their political goals of unlimited abortion. And other medical organizations that should be objective and nonpartisan, like the National Cancer Institute (NCI), have chosen to ignore the data or put out bromides that don't acknowledge the evidence that exists. But what is important—as one federal judge said in another medical context—"is what the studies show and not what some organization says about the studies."[14]

We look, therefore, to the growing number of international studies from numerous countries that research abortion and its impact on women, focusing on three long-term impacts: abortion and breast cancer, abortion and pre-term birth, and abortion and mental health risks.

Abortion and Breast Cancer

Breast cancer is a leading cause of death for women ages 20–59, and the severity and incident rate are getting worse. In recent decades, researchers have observed that women ages 25–39 are getting advanced breast cancer that is more aggressive than ever before. And incidence of breast cancer is higher today than it was a generation ago: in 1970, one in twelve women experienced breast cancer; by 2016, it was one in eight. The increased incidence of breast cancer over the past four decades has coincided with the increase in elective abortion.

Decades ago, medical researchers found a reasonable biological connection between abortion and breast cancer. We can understand the plausible association between abortion and breast cancer by examining the physiology of the breast and the interaction of pregnancy and breast tissue.

At full development, the breast is comprised of between fifteen and twenty segments, called lobes, which are made up of lobules. There are four stages of breast tissue development, with four corresponding types of lobules, Types 1–4. Ductal breast cancer, which represents 85 percent of all breast cancers, starts in lobule Type 1. Lobular breast cancer, which represents another 12 percent of all breast cancers, starts in lobule Type 2. Lobule Type 4 is cancer resistant, as is Type 3 when Type 4 lobules have regressed post-birth.

During the course of regular monthly hormone shifts, Type 1 lobules naturally mature into Type 2. During pregnancy, there are even more of them. With the onset of pregnancy, hormone levels are immediately elevated; the embryo—even before implantation—produces human chorionic gonadotropin (hCG). When that hormone increases, it stimulates the ovaries to produce more estrogen and progesterone, which in turn stimulates the woman's breast tissue to grow. In early pregnancy, then, the woman's breast tissue is vulnerable to cancer because her breast tissue is making Type 1 and 2 lobules and there are more places for cancer to start.

Once the pregnancy is carried to term, the risk subsides due to the protective effect of full-term pregnancy. In a typical pregnancy, after 32 weeks, the human placental lactogen (hPL) increases, which results in full differentiation of her breast tissue to lobule Type 4 and the full, long-lasting protective effect of a full-term pregnancy against breast cancer.

That normal, healthy process is abruptly stopped by the artificial termination of pregnancy. When the pregnancy is terminated before that full differentiation process, the breast tissue is more vulnerable to cancer due to its exposure to estrogen and subsequent growth in Types 1 and 2 lobules without allowing them to progress to cancer-resistant Type 4 lobules. This has been confirmed by the research of Jose Russo and Irma Russo,[15] and by the testimony of a leading French medical oncologist, Dr. Pierre Band.[16]

This biological plausibility of the association between elective abortion and breast cancer is supported by some statistical research. As of 2016, there were 108 worldwide studies on the association. There is a diversity in the findings of these studies; some show an increased risk of breast cancer after abortion, and some show a decreased risk. But overall, of the 108 worldwide studies examining women from many different countries, 56 found a strong link between abortion and breast cancer, 23 found a lesser link, and 29 found no link at all.

Though studies finding an association go back to 1957, perhaps the first major such study was published in 1994 by Dr. Janet Daling in the *Journal of the National Cancer Institute* (NCI), a part of the National Institutes of Health (NIH). Daling found a significantly increased risk of breast cancer after abortion. Specifically, Daling concluded, "Among women who had been pregnant at least once, the risk of breast cancer in those who had experienced an induced abortion was 50% higher than among other women."[17]

Two years after the Daling study, Dr. Joel Brind and colleagues published a meta-analysis reviewing and reexamining 23 studies in the *Journal of Epidemiology and Community Health*. They found a 30 percent increased risk of breast cancer for women with abortion histories.[18]

Yet despite what is known about the physiology of the breast, the acknowledged increase in breast cancer risk from delaying a first full-term pregnancy (FFTP), and the cumulative findings of the 108 studies that have been conducted, the abortion-breast cancer association has been summarily dismissed by influential OB-GYN authorities. And when the producer of the 2016 documentary *Hush* tried to interview major medical organizations on the abortion-breast cancer link, all denied an interview.[19] They simply said that the case was closed. Despite the 108 studies existing in 2016, there has been no further response from the NCI.

How is this justified? Each of the major medical organizations that dismisses an association between abortion and breast cancer relies on a brief 2003 workshop sponsored by the National Cancer Institute (NCI) of the National Institutes of Health (NIH) in Bethesda, Maryland. Only one brief paper on the association between elective abortion and breast cancer was presented at the workshop; in it, Dr. Leslie Bernstein addressed conclusions since Brind's 1996 meta-analysis. After a brief review of the existing studies, Bernstein issued a broad, sweeping statement: that they "show no adverse impact of induced abortion or miscarriage on breast cancer risk."[20] Dr. Patrick Fagan, who coauthored a 2014 review of the existing studies, believes, "over time, that 2003 conference will become an embarrassment in the history of the NCI."[21]

Abortion and Pre-Term Birth

Women also need to be informed about the studies and findings on the association between abortion and pre-term birth (PTB). Every year, 500,000 babies are born preterm in the United States—one of the highest PTB rates in the world—and over 11,000 die. Doctors have noted that the PTB rate in the US doubled between 1970 (6.6%) and 2006 (12.6%).[22]

Surgical abortion may be associated with PTB because surgical abortion requires the cervix to be artificially enlarged with instruments, which may carry the risk of weakening it. It is known that a certain percentage of women will experience cervical incompetence after abortion, leading to placenta previa and premature or unsuccessful birth.

More than eighty studies, including a strong 2009 study by P. S. Shah, have found an increased risk for PTB after elective abortion. That risk is increased after multiple abortions.[23]

However, similar to the 2003 NIH workshop on abortion and breast cancer, the US Surgeon General sponsored a 2008 workshop on the prevention of pre-term birth. Despite the many existing studies that have found an increased risk of PTB after abortion, the leaders of that workshop refused to allow discussion of the possible link between elective abortion and PTB.

Abortion and Mental Trauma

Women must also be informed about the studies on the association between mental health concerns and abortion. While studies of the association between abortion and mental trauma yield diverse findings, we must note that much of the research is tainted by selection bias, including women not wanting to participate in the studies and other concerns, as I discussed in my *Washington Examiner* op-ed, "What a Flawed Study Ignores about Abortion Regrets."[24] The overwhelming majority of women who choose not to be part of a study are those most likely to have experienced the strongest emotions and regret after their abortion. Conversely, the women who do choose to be a part of research are the most comfortable with and eager to talk about abortion—and are thus the least likely to regret their decision. Certainly, women have different experiences, and not all women will experience trauma. But it is important to follow women for an extended period of time to have accurate findings. And a significant percentage find, over time, that the abortion harmed them more than it helped.

A 2011 study, authored by researcher Priscilla Coleman and published in the *British Journal of Psychiatry*, analyzed close to 900,000 women and found that women who had an abortion had a higher risk of negative outcomes than women who delivered an unintended pregnancy; "women who had undergone an abortion experienced an 81 percent increased risk of mental health problems," including substance abuse, suicidal behavior, depression, and anxiety, and "nearly 10 percent of the incidence of mental health problems was shown to be attributable to abortion." The study found women who have had an abortion are 34 percent more likely to develop an anxiety disorder and 37 percent more likely to experience depression.[25]

While a 2008 task force by the American Psychological Association (APA) found that among adult women who have a legal first-trimester abortion of a single pregnancy, subsequent mental health problems are no greater than among women giving birth, the APA did admit that there are fourteen risk factors increasing the likelihood for women to suffer post-abortion psychological problems. These include being pressured into the abortion, having had more than one abortion, or having an abortion during adolescence.[26]

Much of the above data on the risks of abortion is discussed in the 2016 must-see documentary *Hush*. It is the best existing presentation of the medical studies on the long-term risks of abortion. This data needs to be reviewed by every woman—and by every minor girl and her parent—before she undergoes an elective abortion.

The Road to *Roe*'s Reversal

So why is *Roe*—this tragic, unconstitutional, disastrous decision—still the law of the land? It reflects the incredible political power and financial resources of abortion advocates that *Roe* has not fallen despite these weaknesses and negative results. But the good news is that *Roe* remains unsettled today despite all the efforts by cultural, political, and legal elites to prop it up.

Our politics, state legislatures, and political commentary show that millions of Americans anticipate that, sooner or later, *Roe* will be overturned. That was clearly demonstrated by the actions of some of the deepest red and blue states in the 2019 state legislative sessions, many of which sought either to outlaw abortion and protect women and children from its harms, or to enshrine abortion on demand into state law.

Roe remains unsettled because it is fatally flawed and subject to constant criticism, and expectations are growing that it will be overturned sooner or later.

Now, despite being radically unsettled, *Roe* won't fall of its own weight because there are numerous, powerful forces in American society working 24/7 to save it. But make no mistake, *Roe* is destined for the dustbin of history.

On the Side of Women

It is important for Americans who stand for life to be on the side of women—intentionally, consistently, and visibly. The life of the child in the womb is not the only moral issue involved in abortion. It is also a moral problem when a woman isn't fully informed about the biological nature of her child or about the risks to her own health.

Fully informed consent is a moral issue—and it is a moral problem when women are pressured into abortion.

The cause for life in America started providing counseling and resources to women with a "crisis pregnancy" in the 1960s. One of the great strengths of the pro-life movement in America is the network of pregnancy care centers across the country—approximately 3,000—that provide direct services to women and their children. From my time as board chair of a pregnancy care center in Maryland, I know just how committed the staff and volunteers are, and the good work they do.

But there is still much to be done. Every church should adopt a pregnancy care center, supporting the staff and the women who seek their services. As suggested by the growing network of pregnancy centers across the fifty states and the tens of millions of dollars raised annually to support those centers, enabling a woman with an unexpected pregnancy to resist the pressure to get an abortion and to choose a life-affirming alternative is the best way to help women who are scared and may feel alone or pressured into abortion.

Myths That Sustain *Roe*

Despite all the efforts to see the tragedy of *Roe* corrected, a number of myths and misconceptions have served to sustain it. It is our job to fight back with the truth and with public education.

MYTH: Overturning Roe *would immediately make abortion illegal.*

It is widely assumed that "overturning *Roe*" means that the Supreme Court would make abortion illegal. That is incorrect. If *Roe* were overturned today, abortion would still be legal in thirty-five or more states tomorrow, and perhaps in all fifty. When *Roe* is overturned, the states *could* enforce abortion limits that are on the books in the state. But most states don't have enforceable prohibitions on the books before 20 weeks of pregnancy. The only way in which overturning *Roe* would make abortion illegal across the states would be if the Court decided the case based on a Fourteenth Amendment rationale that considered all unborn Americans "persons" entitled to individual constitutional rights. While this direction may be legally sound, it is more likely that the Court may instead simply send the issue of the legality of abortion back to the states, instead of forbidding it across the country.

MYTH: Women would be prosecuted for abortion if Roe *were overturned.*

For a century before *Roe*, state abortion prohibitions targeted doctors or those who induce them, not women. State legislatures and state courts explicitly recognized women as the second "victim" of abortion. The irony is that, instead of states prosecuting women, the exact opposite is true. To protect their own interests, it was abortionists (like the cult hero and abortionist Ruth Barnett when Oregon last prosecuted her in 1968) who, when they were prosecuted, sought to haul into court the women on whom they had performed abortions. As a matter of criminal evidentiary law, if the court treated the woman as an accomplice, she could not testify against the abortionist, and the case against the abortionist would be thrown out.[27]

MYTH: Women need abortion for equal opportunity in America.

No reliable social science data show that women's educational or career success depends on elective abortion. Women are strong and capable, and we don't have to choose between family and career—more than ever before thanks to the many laws that have been passed since *Roe* to provide pregnancy and parenting protections. And social science data indicate that if women and men rely on anything to level the playing field in a nation that has not yet achieved equal opportunities for parents, it is contraceptives, not abortion.

The Supreme Court's June 2020 Abortion Decision

The Court's June 2020 abortion decision in *June Medical Services v. Russo* was widely misreported in the press and therefore has been misunderstood by the public. But it settled nothing; in fact, it kept *Roe unsettled* by changing, once again, the rules of the game.[28]

Chief Justice John Roberts did vote with the four pro-abortion justices to invalidate the Louisiana law that required abortionists to have "admitting privileges" at a local hospital to smoothly transfer and admit women who suffer complications from abortion—to give them every chance at getting lifesaving care. It is a women's rights issue; the decision handed a legal loophole to abortion businesses and left Louisiana women who seek abortions as second-class citizens. But there is much more to the story.

After applying a 2016 decision from Texas to strike down the Louisiana law on the basis of precedent, Chief Justice Roberts then repudiated the Court's ruling and turned around and joined with the other four "conservative" justices to indicate that he would apply more lenient standards to review state abortion limits in the future. By adding his fifth voice to the other four, they effectively undermined that 2016 decision from Texas.

Four justices issued strong dissents. Justice Clarence Thomas said he would throw out the Court's abortion decisions entirely. Justice Samuel Alito wrote a strong dissent, joined by Justices Thomas, Gorsuch, and Kavanaugh, explaining that the evidence showed the Louisiana law would serve to protect women's health. Justice

Kavanaugh joined that opinion. And Justice Gorsuch dissented and questioned the Court's abortion doctrine.

So despite the vote going in favor of the pro-abortion justices, *June Medical* coalesced a new majority that said they would apply more lenient standards to state abortion limits in the future.

The Need for a Sixth Justice

It has been clear that we needed a sixth justice to create a larger majority before the Court might be willing to reconsider *Roe v. Wade*. With the elevation of Justice Amy Coney Barrett to the Supreme Court bench, we may have that sixth justice. We know that she looks to the constitution, rather than to personal preference, when ruling on difficult cases.

There is inherent value and importance in having the largest possible majority of the nine Justices to join in overturning *Roe*. A 5–4 overruling would be inherently unstable. A pro-abortion president could, for example, name a replacement for one of the *June Medical* five, and the overruling might be overturned.

We have seen this in prior decisions that were politically controversial and had national impact, for example on the issue of racial segregation. In 1896, in *Plessy v. Ferguson*, the Supreme Court created the "separate but equal" doctrine to uphold the constitutionality of segregation—another time that the Court dehumanized and discriminated against a broad class of human beings who lacked adequate representation based on an inherent trait. In 1953, however, Earl Warren was seated as Chief Justice of the Supreme Court, where he worked patiently, month after month, to form a unanimous Court around an opinion that would overturn racial segregation. In 1954, fifty-eight years after *Plessy*, his efforts bore fruit with the *Brown v.*

Board of Education decision, in which the justices ruled unanimously that racial segregation of children in public schools is unconstitutional. The efforts to overturn *Roe* may well follow that precedent.

The Critical Role of Elections

This highlights the critical role that elections will likewise play in the future of *Roe*. In the American constitutional system, the federal courts are shaped by the politically accountable branches. The president nominates and the Senate confirms—or not—as we saw when Justice Scalia died in February 2016 and the Senate majority leader immediately announced that no hearings would be held on any nominee before the November election. The makeup of the Supreme Court, then, is directly determined by presidential and senatorial elections, and as critical and consequential as the work in the states is as we strive to restore respect for life, we must not neglect our national elections, which can have generational consequences.

Conclusion

Roe v. Wade is a tragic, self-inflicted wound by the Supreme Court that must be corrected. It is unsettled because the cause for life in America has kept it unsettled over decades by legal, political, and social opposition. It would be good for the country and for the Court to overturn *Roe*, thereby decentralizing the issue and returning the abortion issue to the people in the States.

The case against *Roe* must continue, month by month, year by year. Pro-life Americans need to persevere, through thick and thin. We owe it to women and their children. We owe it to our daughters and our granddaughters, and generations yet unborn.

I am confident that one day soon *Roe* will be relegated to the dustbin of history alongside other disgraceful precedents like *Dred Scott v. Sandford*. We will continue to prosecute the case until all children are welcomed in life and protected in law.

CLAIM 2

The Fetus Is Not a Person

3

Made in God's Image: Personhood according to Scripture

—Jeanette Hagen Pifer—

What is man that you are mindful of him,
and the son of man that you care for him?
Yet you have made him a little lower than the heavenly beings
and crowned him with glory and honor.
Psalm 8:4–5

In worship of God's majesty, and in view of His magnificent creation, David asks a penetrating question: Why is it that God cares so profoundly for the human race? Why has God given such an elevated standing to humankind? Throughout Scripture we find a unique status given to God's human creation: humans were purposed to reflect the glory of the Lord within the created realm in unique ways. With such divine intention, it follows that one of the clearest prohibitions within the Ten Commandments is Exodus 20:13: "You shall not murder." One human shall not interfere with God's sovereign design over another human. In the context of the abortion debate, much ink has been spilled, and many heated arguments have arisen, over the question of the status of the unborn. Is that which is growing and developing inside a woman's uterus a *person*? And thus, does this commandment apply to taking the life of the unborn?

In this section of the book, we will be exploring the pro-choice claim that the fetus is not a person. For many pro-choice proponents, the fetus is a glob of tissue. Others understand that there is profound biological development taking place from the moment of conception, but they argue that the special status of personhood should not be granted until birth. We will tackle this issue from four different angles: the Bible, philosophy, biology, and law. Solid arguments in favor of the personhood of the fetus from philosophical, biological, and legal perspectives are imperative in debates with non-Christians. For believers, we have the added benefit of considering God's heart on the issue as we seek to understand the concept of personhood as revealed in Scripture. Because the Bible is the Christian's source of ultimate truth (Ps. 119:160; Prov. 30:5), it will be important to ground the personhood of the fetus biblically when in conversation with believers.

In pursuing this study, we must be up front about the fact that the Bible does not speak explicitly of the personhood of the developing baby, nor is the issue of abortion dealt with directly in Scripture. However, there is evidence that prenatal life was viewed with as much value as postnatal life by the biblical authors. This chapter will begin by offering a definition of personhood rooted in the biblical concept of being made in God's image, which in itself has major implications for the sanctity of life, both born and unborn. We will then look at specific texts in which prenatal life is explicitly addressed in order to discover whether the concept of personhood can be applied to these early stages of development. Through our study, we will discover that there is a strong biblical case to be made for the personhood of the fetus and, more importantly, we will uncover God's sovereign design over, intimate knowledge of, and parental care for His precious ones in the earliest stages of life. This biblical basis should ground our conviction all the more in the fight to save the lives of unborn babies.

Defining Personhood

To begin, we must do our best to define our terms. If we are speaking of the "personhood" of an embryo or fetus, what exactly do we mean by "person"? Calum MacKellar explains that there never was a clear understanding of personhood in the ancient world.[1] In our modern context, there are vast and varied understandings of personhood as well. Some Western notions characterize personhood in terms of being a self-conscious and rational being, and thus a person is defined based on whether and to what extent one is able to express his or her rational nature.[2] This ultimately reduces personhood to what someone can *do*, which is problematic for a number of reasons. First, leaving aside the question of the personhood of the embryo, this implies that the status of personhood may cease to be applied to some individuals before their body actually dies. Furthermore, it implies that the personhood of an individual could increase or decrease in correspondence with his or her ability to convey rationality.

This understanding of personhood is widely challenged, since specific abilities and characteristics are secondary and do not have to be displayed at every moment in life for that individual to have value. MacKellar clarifies the issue: "Having a rational nature . . . does not mean that rationality must always be present. . . . What is important is having the constitution of beings of a human kind, rather than being able to express such a nature."[3] Thus, an unconscious adult continues to be a person even though the ability to display rationality may cease temporarily (e.g., during sleep) or even permanently (e.g., in comatose).

While a lack of a clear understanding of personhood has persisted in secular thought, theological reflection within the church has provided much-needed clarity. As the early church fathers contemplated the radical distinction between the Creator God and His creation, more attention was given to defining the nature of individuals within the created realm. Theologian John Zizioulas points out: "Although the person and 'personal identity' are widely discussed nowadays as a supreme ideal, nobody seems to recognize that historically as well as existentially the concept of the person is indissolubly bound up with theology."[4] Indeed, from a theological perspective, human personal identity must connect in some way to the personal nature of God. More specifically, MacKellar has defined a person in this way: "a being with a full inherent dignity reflecting the image of God."[5] This will be our working definition of personhood in this chapter.

The Sacred Creation of Humankind

If personhood is centered on the idea of "reflecting the image of God," it makes sense to begin exploring the biblical concept of personhood in the creation story, the beginning of God's revelatory program. The remainder of the biblical witness, and indeed all of Christian theology, is grounded on the creation narrative, which announces two foundational truths. First, it reveals *who God is* in relation to the cosmos, to the natural order, and to humanity—He is the sovereign Creator and majestic Lord of the universe and of all creation, both human and non-human.[6] Second, the creation narrative reveals *what humanity is* and what distinguishes it from the rest of God's handiwork. Here we focus on this second question, and our answers are found right in Genesis 1–2. There we learn that Adam (representing all humanity) was not just another animal or thing among many other parts of creation, but was dignified above the rest of the created order. Humanity represents the pinnacle of God's creation, possesses a special identity and relation to God, and is therefore to be protected.[7]

The Image of God

We are first introduced to the "image of God" in Genesis 1:26, where God announces: "Let us make man in our *image*, after our *likeness*." Every word in this statement is important, though space only allows us to focus on a couple of key terms. First, the Hebrew word for "man" (*adam*), although sometimes referring to individuals, predominantly refers to the entire class of humanity and can thus be translated as "humankind."[8] Second, the idea of "our likeness" reiterates and highlights the preceding expression, "our image."[9] But what precisely does it mean to possess *God's image*?

On the one hand, the immediately following verses in Genesis illuminate the *purpose* of being made in God's image—humanity, who was charged to "be fruitful and multiply and fill the earth," was made in God's image so that they would "have dominion" over every living thing on the earth (Gen. 1:28, 26). The charge to exercise dominion fits with what is known about how regal imaging was practiced in the Ancient Near East. Gerhard von Rad, for example, noted: "Just as powerful earthly kings, to indicate their claim to dominion, erect an image of themselves in the provinces of their empire where they do not personally appear, so man is placed upon earth in God's image as God's sovereign emblem."[10] The idea is that God placed humanity into His creation in order to represent Him on earth. This also fits with the meaning of the Hebrew term for "image" (*selem*), which conveys the idea of a representation of something by a picture, statue, relief, or drawing.[11] As God's statue, living and working among the rest of creation, the purpose of humanity is to represent God's authority and purposes—to stand in place of Him.

On the other hand, being made in the image of God also has implications for how we understand the nature of human identity, which can only be known by understanding God. Robert Saucy elucidates: "For that which is by nature the 'image' of something else can only be fully understood by knowing that which it images."[12] On this basis we discover the most significant aspect of being human: "The human being is a personal individual known and loved by God."[13] Paul affirms that human identity comes from God alone, as recorded in Acts 17:28: "In him we live and move and have our being." That humans were created to have a relationship with their Maker makes them distinct from every other aspect of creation, and this forms the basis of human personal identity.[14]

Equipped with this understanding of the image of God, we can begin to understand the relevance of the creation narrative to our topic of the personhood of the fetus. If God made man in His own image, and *man* refers to everyone belonging to the human species, then the image of God belongs to the born and unborn alike—even to the embryo and to the fetus. As we will see in the chapter on personhood according to biology, humanity is not determined by gestational age, but by having the genetic composition of the human race. Indeed, all human life is sacredly designed by God, purposed to reflect His glory and to exist in relationship to Him. Thus, it is because humans possess this special aspect of God's identity that He demands that all human life be protected. As God declares to Noah's family later in the Genesis narrative, after charging them to repopulate the earth:

> "Whoever sheds the blood of man,
> by man shall his blood be shed,
> for God made man in his own image." (Gen. 9:6)

In this important verse, God prohibits the killing of fellow human beings *by virtue of the fact that they possess God's image*. This prohibition unquestionably applies to preborn humans just as much as it does to those who have been birthed. But the above verses in Genesis are not alone in Scripture in their validation of the personhood of the unborn. As we will see in the next section, this *relational dynamic of bearing God's image* is evident in texts across the Bible that address the child in utero.

The Personal Nature of Life in the Womb

Let us now examine some other key texts that help us answer our question of whether the Bible attributes the status of personhood to the unborn. It will be important to demonstrate that the same characteristics are ascribed to the unborn as to a person outside of the womb. Furthermore, it will be important to examine God's perspective—how does God view what occurs in the earliest stages of embryonic and fetal development? Is there evidence that the concept of the relational "image of God" is applied in these passages?

Do we see evidence of His sovereign design, His loving care, and personal involvement at such nascent stages?

We begin in the Old Testament, in the book of Job. After experiencing a series of severe trials, Job laments:

> "Let the day perish on which I was born,
> And the night that said, 'A man is conceived.'" (Job 3:3)

Here the writer employs parallelism, a common Hebrew poetic device in which the second line corresponds in some way to the idea expressed in the first. In this text, Job declares that which is conceived belongs on the same developmental spectrum as "a man" (*gever*). Later, Job continues his lament by questioning:

> "Why did I not die at birth,
> come out from the womb and expire?" (Job 3:11)

The very possibility that Job could "die at birth" suggests that being born is but a continuation of the life that began at conception, a life separate from the mother's own life.

This continuity between conception and birth is seen in several other passages in the Old Testament, many of which reveal God's perception of the fetus—that is, God involves Himself in personally calling, caring for, and sovereignly designing life at its earliest stages. For example, in Jeremiah 1:5 God states:

> "Before I formed you in the womb I knew you, and before you were born I consecrated you; I have appointed you a prophet to the nations."

In this famous commissioning text, God reveals that He knew Jeremiah intimately even in the womb, and this was in some way the same kind of relational knowledge He had of Jeremiah while he served in prophetic ministry as an adult. His calling to be a prophet was established while in the womb, a status that was usually given to prophets in their adulthood. Furthermore, this calling was of a personal and relational nature—something that makes sense only if the preborn Jeremiah was in fact a person.

We find another example of the Lord's intimate, prenatal knowledge and appointment of a prophet in Isaiah 49:1:

> "The Lord called me from the womb, from the body of my mother he named my name."

Again, the Lord calls and names Isaiah even from his mother's womb and at some unspecified moment during his mother's pregnancy. This activity depicts the kind of relational interest we see God taking in persons outside the womb—something that is nonsensical if that which the mother carries inside of her is "merely a blob of tissue."[15]

Psalm 139:13–16 provides one of the most well-known and important proofs that God intimately knows and loves the unborn.

> For you formed my inward parts;
>   you knitted me together in my mother's womb.
> I praise you, for I am fearfully and wonderfully made.
> Wonderful are your works;
>   my soul knows it very well.
> My frame was not hidden from you,
> when I was being made in secret,
>   intricately woven in the depths of the earth.

> Your eyes saw my unformed substance;
> in your book were written, every one of them,
> the days that were formed for me,
> when as yet there was none of them.

This beautiful picture of God's sovereign design and intimate knowledge of the unborn child speaks volumes about the sanctity of life that is divinely developed inside the womb. Some contend that the psalmist only refers to the development of a being that *eventually becomes* a person. However, as Scott Rae argues in chapter 4, a human being does not develop from a being that is *not* human. Within this passage we find indications of the *continuity of personhood* that is described from the early gestational stages within the womb to adulthood. The psalmist who describes the intimate knowledge God has of him as an adult is the same person who is so "intricately woven" by God in utero (Ps. 139:15).[16] It is clear that what is depicted in the womb is the same person who eventually writes this familiar psalm.

In verse 16, the Hebrew word for "unformed substance," or in some translations, "unformed body," is *golem*. Some Hebrew lexicons translate this as "embryo."[17] Thus, from the earliest gestational stages that which is developing inside his or her mother is seen, designed, and cherished by God. Old Testament scholar John Goldingay points out that the wonder this psalm "expresses at the growth of a fetus and at Yhwh's involvement in this process is grounds for reckoning that a decision to cause a woman to miscarry is not merely one involving a decision about what happens to her body. It involves terminating a project that Yhwh is involved in."[18]

The "eyes of God" in verse 16 are also significant. Throughout the Bible, mention of God's eyes or God "seeing" signifies something beyond normal human knowledge or awareness, but more intimately suggests God's care, concern, and blessing. For example, in Psalm 101:6 God's eyes look on the faithful in the land with favor. In 1 Kings 9:3, God promises that His eyes and heart will be on the temple for all time. And in Numbers 6:24–25, we find the famous and oft-bestowed Aaronic blessing: "The LORD bless you and keep you; the LORD make his face to shine upon you and be gracious to you." These examples suggest that in Psalm 139:16, God's eyes convey His personal concern for and relationship with David, even while in utero. John Davis confirms that this passage elucidates for us "from God's eye point of view the wonder of the intrauterine development of the embryonic human. It is abundantly clear that God, the divine 'parent' has already 'bonded' with the child he is making."[19] All of God's sovereignty, personal concern, and care for humanity are abundantly evident in this depiction of life, even from the point of conception.

Moving now to the New Testament, one of the most significant texts in support of prenatal personhood is found in the announcement of the conception of the Christ. Luke 1:26–56 tells the miraculous story of the incarnation. The angel Gabriel announced to Mary that she would conceive by the power of the Holy Spirit: "The Holy Spirit will come upon you, and the power of the Most High will overshadow you; therefore the child to be born will be called holy—the Son of God" (Luke 1:35). A couple of significant observations can be made when Mary visits her cousin, Elizabeth, just days after this announcement. First, Elizabeth's baby leaped in her womb (Luke 1:41), indicating a living being that was responding to the life within Mary, even at the embryonic stage.[20] Second, Elizabeth proclaims that Mary is the "mother" of her Lord (Luke 1:43), which suggests that Elizabeth, as well as Luke the narrator, believed what Mary was carrying was in fact a child, not just tissue.

Altogether, what we can conclude from this passage is that the incarnation occurred from the moment of conception. Jesus did not *become* the uniquely divine and human person after He was born, or when He was twelve years old speaking with the teachers in the temple, or as an adult ministering to the multitudes. Personhood was attributed to Jesus from the moment He was miraculously conceived in the womb of Mary. Indeed, she was instructed to view the miracle that occurred within her in very personal terms. Jesus was identified as her son and given a personal name, Jesus. Davis elucidates the implications of these details: "There is no place here for some impersonal biological terminology of the 'products of conception.' The divine 'speech-act' mediated by Gabriel confers personal status on Jesus in his embryonic state."[21] Indeed, the incarnation of Jesus attests to the sanctity of prenatal life: "His human history, like ours, began at conception. . . . The significant point is that God chose to begin the process of incarnation there, rather than at some other point, thus affirming the significance of that starting point for human life."[22]

The Protection of Prenatal Life in Ancient Israel

There is one passage of Scripture that clearly shows God's attitude toward the protection of the unborn—indeed, one that explicitly addresses how God's people were to handle cases wherein prenatal life was at risk—Exodus 21:22–25. Because this passage involves activity that jeopardizes the life of a human fetus, it is often appealed to in the abortion debate.

Exodus 21:22–25 is an example of case law in Israel's legal code. In such cases, a condition is introduced ("if/when . . . "), which is then followed by a penalty ("then . . . "). This particular case addresses how to handle situations involving a pregnant woman in which "harm" is caused.

> When men strive together and hit a pregnant woman, so that her children come out, but there is no harm, the one who hit her shall surely be fined, as the woman's husband shall impose on him, and he shall pay as the judges determine. But if there is harm, then you shall pay life for life, eye for eye, tooth for tooth, hand for hand, foot for foot, burn for burn, wound for wound, stripe for stripe.

This passage presents two different scenarios: (A) a pregnant woman is struck so that "her child comes out,"[23] no harm is caused, and a fine is owed by the man who hit her; (B) a pregnant woman is struck, harm is caused, and thus the guilty party is given the more serious sentence of "life for life, eye for eye," and so on. This text has actually been used by both pro-choice and pro-life advocates to justify their stance. That two sides can use one text to support their opposing views is due to a few translation difficulties, which we will work through in order to discern the best reading of the passage.

The first issue to tackle is how to translate the Hebrew verb *yatsa*. The verb means "to come out" or to "go out" and is translated in this literal way in many English versions (English Standard Version, Lexham English Bible, New Century Version). Since "to come out" is somewhat vague, other translations have interpreted this either as a live, premature birth, or as a miscarriage. Only the Revised and New Revised Standard Versions (RSV, NRSV) translate this as miscarriage, but a significant number of scholars hold to this translation.[24] However, there are sufficient reasons to doubt that miscarriage is in view in Exodus 21:22. First, *yatsa* is not the normal word for miscarriage used in the Old Testament. There are two other Hebrew words used unmistakably to refer to a miscarriage. First, the word *nefel* is used in Psalm 58:8, Job 3:16, and Ecclesiastes 6:3 (translated as either miscarriage or stillborn child).[25] The Old Testament also uses variations of the root *shkl,* for example, in Exodus 23:26 and Hosea 9:14.[26] Use of either of these verbs would indicate that the baby was born dead. The fact that neither of these explicit references to miscarriage is used casts reasonable doubt on whether Exodus 21:22 refers to the death of the fetus.

A better understanding of the meaning of the word used in Exodus 21:22 is "premature birth" and is based on semantics, biblical context, and syntax. On semantic grounds, the verb conveys the transition of the fetus from inside the mother's womb to the outside, and does not in itself provide any indications of the baby's condition.[27] However, additional insight can be gleaned from its usage elsewhere in the Old Testament. In the sixteen times this verb is used to describe giving birth, fifteen cases record a successful delivery, although many times in abnormal and challenging situations.[28] To offer a couple of examples, the verb is used to recount the successful births of two sets of twins: Jacob and Esau, and Zerah and Perez (Gen. 25:22–26; 38:27–30). Twin pregnancies are considered high risk even in modern medicine; how much more would the risk have been in these primitive accounts? Yet, in both instances, the twins "came out" healthy. A number of other occurrences of *yatsa* that resulted in the births of healthy babies could be cited, but the point is that the biblical texts generally employ this verb to convey a premature birth, and often under some kind of duress.[29] Only in Numbers 12:12 do we see a case that did not result in a live birth. Here the result is a stillbirth, but this is not implied through the verb *yatsa*—rather, it is indicated through the addition of the verb *muth* ("to die") at the beginning of the verse.[30] Thus, if all of the texts in the Pentateuch that employ *yatsa* without modification do so in live-birth scenarios, it makes sense to assume the same is the case in Exodus 21:22. On the basis of semantic grounds and biblical context, a live, "premature" birth finds the most support.

Another translation issue falls on syntactical grounds: how should we understand the qualifying clauses, "there is no harm," and "there is harm"? Do these apply to the mother, to the child, or to both? More specifically, do these modify the child coming out of the womb, so that in the first instance the child, although premature, is born healthy, and in the second instance, the child suffers either injury or death?[31] Those who understand verse 22 to describe a miscarriage assume that harm had already been done to the fetus, and thus they must add the word "further" or "other" before "harm" in verses 22–23 to indicate whether or not harm was done specifically to the mother. However, "further" or "other" do not appear in the original Hebrew. In fact, the word "harm" appears immediately after the clause "her children come out," and is indefinite, implying that it refers at least to the premature baby and is probably inclusive of the mother as well.[32] As qualifiers, the two phrases complete the description of the child's premature birth—indicating whether or not the birth involved injury or death.

In light of these semantical, contextual, and syntactical grounds, there is good reason to interpret the legal case presented in Exodus 21:22–25 as involving a premature, live birth. The expressions "with/without harm" refer to both mother and child. Thus, in scenario A, where there is no harm done to either mother or child, the less severe consequence of a fine is due. However, in scenario B, where there is harm done to the child, and possibly also to the mother, the *lex taliones*—law of retaliation ("eye for eye, tooth for tooth," etc.)—is applicable. The person who has injured another person is to be penalized to the same degree as the harm they inflicted on others. This passage, frequently misapplied by pro-choice proponents, accords more consistently with the pro-life position. Indeed, it demonstrates that from the very inception of Israel as a nation, prenatal life was not only valued but protected in God's covenant law.

Conclusion

From the beginning of Genesis and throughout the Bible, we see that God has dignified His human creation—as His image bearers, humans possess special identity and relation to God. In the biblical texts we examined, it is evident that from God's perspective, there is a continuity of personal identity from inside to outside the womb. In each passage explored in this chapter, and several more, we see that personal characteristics are ascribed to the preborn.[33] From God's calling of Jeremiah and Isaiah, to His intimate knowledge of David, to the incarnation of Jesus Christ—the uniquely divine and human Son of God—we see confirmation that embryos and fetuses are lives with inherent worth and capacity for relationship with their Maker. Davis notes: "The effect of such texts is to 'personalize' the unborn" and thus we are enabled to view the "embryonic human being from a 'God's-eye' point of view."[34] Indeed, this "God's eye" point of view reveals His sovereign design, His loving care, and personal protection over the earliest nascent stages of life.

So, in answer to our initial questions, the scriptural witness portrays *that which is growing and developing inside a woman's uterus as a person*—indeed, an image bearer of God, and the commandment not to murder absolutely applies to taking the life of the unborn.

4

More Than the Sum of Its Parts: Philosophical Reflections on Human Personhood

—Scott B. Rae—

Most of the critical issues in bioethics today revolve around a central question—what constitutes a human person? Or to put it another way, who counts as a member of the human community? For some time, this question has been central to the cultural debate on abortion. For pro-life advocates, it is considered *the* main question, really the only question that matters, and the answer to it determines one's position on abortion definitively. For if the unborn is a person with the right to life, that settles the morality of abortion. But if not, that opens the door to abortion, as well as destruction of embryos as moral options. However, increasingly some pro-choice advocates are conceding that the unborn are full persons, and yet making an abortion rights argument all the same. The pro-life advocate has unwittingly "upped the ante" once that concession is made, by insisting that not only does the unborn have the right to life, but he or she also has a claim on the mother's body for the resources needed to survive and flourish. The position most consistent with Scripture is known in philosophical terms as a *substance view* of a human person, which I will outline and defend in this chapter.

Substances and Property-Things

A properly grounded philosophical view of human persons involves making a key distinction between two different types of entities, *substances* and *property-things*.[1] Living things such as plants, animals, and human beings are examples of substances, while inanimate objects such as cars and machinery are examples of property things. The difference is that a substance has an internal essence that defines it and orders its change and development according to observable principles. A substance is an entity in which the whole is greater than the sum of its parts, and the whole contains the essence, or internal ordering principle that gives it its unity and cohesiveness. By contrast, a property-thing is no more than an ordered aggregate of its parts. It is ordered, but the order is externally imposed and there is no internal defining essence or principle that directs its change and development, nor is there any essence that informs and unifies its parts and properties. It is merely a collection of parts, standing in external space and time relations that, in turn, gives rise to a bundle of externally related properties that are determined by those parts.

The same is not true with a substance, for example, a dog. The properties of a dog are different from the properties of an automobile. The properties of the dog are grounded in, unified by, and emerge from the dog's essence. That is, a dog is the way it is because it possesses an internal essence that defines and orders its properties. Thus, a dog is more than the external organization of its parts functioning in a given way. Its properties are deeply unified and related internally as part of the essential nature of "dogness." A dog is what it is apart from social convention, and its properties exist only in the context of a coherent, ontological whole. By contrast, a car has no essence beyond its parts. Those parts are bundled together to form a loosely unified whole. Since a car has no internal essence or nature, an ordering principle is externally imposed upon a set of parts to form a bundle of properties by human convention. In this case, engineers put the parts of the car together according to a blueprint that another set of engineers drafted. The order and structure of the car are imposed entirely from without, in contrast to a dog, whose order and structure emerge from within, from its nature. To possess an internal nature, then, is possible only for substances. Their essential nature informs their being and gives them the essential properties that are characteristic of their natural kind. All members of a given species express the same essential nature, though there are differences in what are called *accidental properties,* such as the color of a dog and whether or not the dog has spots.

So while substances possess an internal nature, property-things do not. There is no internal, ordering principle or force that is capable of grounding a car's unity, governing its change, or guiding its movement toward any end. Instead, there are only modifications caused by external forces, namely engineers and mechanics who work on the car. Human beings designed and built the automobile by arranging its materials into a specific pattern that would allow the car to function according to their design. The materials that were used to manufacture a car had no inherent inclination to be so structured, and its parts are externally ordered, imposed by forces outside the car itself, namely the assembly line workers who assembled the car. Each of the materials used to build the car could have been used to make a variety of other things, by arranging them in different designs. For example, the tires could be used for a variety of other vehicles, and the metal that makes up many of the engine parts could be used for countless other metal objects. It just so happened that the external forces, that is, the design of the engineers and assemblers, arranged these parts into a car. There was nothing intrinsic to the car that demanded that its parts be ordered like they are.

By contrast, a puppy matures into an adult dog, and an acorn matures into an oak tree, according to its internal essence. This essence, or nature, directs the developmental process of the substance and establishes limits on the variations each substance may undergo and still exist. For example, the acorn will not grow into a dog and the dog will not become an oak tree. Consequently, a substance functions in light of what it is, and maintains its essence regardless of the degree to which its ultimate capacities are realized.

While there are variations among the individual members of a class of substances, such as differences in features between a Dalmatian and a golden retriever and, like differences in the stages of development, such variance does not affect the essential nature of their being. For it is the underlying essence of a thing, not its stage of development at a given point, that constitutes what it is. A puppy is not of a different kind than an adult dog, nor is a sapling of a different kind than a full-grown oak tree.

As a substance grows, it does not become more of its kind, nor does it become something altogether different, but rather, it matures according to its kind. The development and realization of its potential, or its capacities, is controlled by the substance's essential nature. The capacities for the acorn one day to develop a trunk, branches, and leaves are already embedded within the acorn, prior to their realization. Whether or not the acorn actually develops into a full-grown oak tree depends on conditions such as its environment and nutrients in the soil. That is, it has capacities that are currently latent and will be expressed if the conditions are right for their development. If they fail to develop, that is the fault of the conditions, not the internal essence or nature. That is, these conditions are independent of the acorn's essential nature. If the conditions are right, it will develop according to its internal design. By contrast, the car has an external design imposed from without that is necessary for it to be assembled into a car.

One helpful distinction between substances and property-things follows from the above discussion. Specifically, substances maintain their identity through change, while property-things do not. The reason for this is that a substance is more than the sum of its parts, which are ordered by some external force. A person can lose a body part such as an appendix, or a dog can shed fur, or an oak tree can lose leaves, and their identity does not change. With each of these substances (persons, dogs, and oak trees), the whole is prior to the parts and these parts have their order because of the internal nature of the substance. By contrast, a property-thing is a collection of its constituent parts. When it loses one of its parts, it technically becomes a different entity. Thus, it cannot maintain its identity over time and through change, because there is no internal ordering essence or principle that grounds its unity. A property-thing becomes a different property-thing when its parts change. No single property-thing can endure through change. It can only undergo a series of changes that result in similar, but ontologically different entities. Though we commonly speak of a car as still being a car if it loses a tire, technically that is not the case. We actually speak of cars as if they were ontologically the same as persons, as though they were both substances. Our common language about cars clearly does not reflect what is metaphysically true about them. Property-things have no enduring essences to ground their identity through change.

Thus, it follows from this distinction that substances maintain their identity through change and property-things do not. To suggest that a human being is a substance, maintaining identity as change occurs, is consistent not only with the biblical teaching that human beings have continuity of personal identity as they mature from embryos/fetuses to adult human beings, but also with our most common ways of speaking about persons and personal identity.

In addition, the common-sense way in which most people view criminal justice and moral responsibility presumes a substance view of a person. Such a view holds that a person remains the same person through time and change. Without such a view of the human person, our common notions of moral and criminal responsibility make little sense. Take for example, a person who commits a violent crime (murder for example, for which there is no statute of limitations for prosecution) and who goes on the run and into hiding for twenty years. At the end of that period, he is captured, taken into custody, and brought to court to face murder charges. Clearly, he has undergone a variety of bodily changes in those twenty years. His mental state may have changed, most of his cells have turned over in that time period, and he may even look like an entirely different person due to physical changes. But imagine if he and his lawyers tried to argue in court that he was a property-thing, not a substance, and as a result, he is a different person from the one who committed the crime twenty years ago. They would conclude that it would be unjust to try him for this crime when a different person actually was the one who committed it. You may think this to be an absurd argument for the person's innocence, and you would be right, and the judge would likely dismiss it out of hand. The reason for both your reaction and the judge's is the presumption that human beings are indeed substances who maintain personal identity through time and change. Our entire concepts of moral responsibility and criminal justice are both premised on this substance view of a person.

Application of a Substance View to the Abortion Debate

The notion of a human being as a substance thus has great significance for the moral status of embryos and fetuses. Virtually everyone accepts that personhood begins at least at birth, though increasingly some argue for the legitimacy of infanticide. Viewing human beings as substances that have continuity of personal identity through time and change strongly suggests that personhood begins at conception. If a human being is indeed a substance, then we could summarize the philosophical argument from substance for the personhood of the unborn, the most controversial of the aspects of personhood, like this. First, an adult human being is the result of the continuous process of growth that begins at conception, about which there is no debate. Second, from conception to adulthood, there is no break in this development which is relevant to the moral status of personhood. Therefore, one is a human being from the point of conception onward, and there is little debate that this conclusion follows from the preceding two premises. The force of this argument clearly rests on the second premise, that there is no morally relevant break in the development from conception to adulthood, though most still agree (advocates of infanticide notwithstanding) that at birth, the newborn child is a full person. Some disagree with this claim, however, and point to certain signposts between conception and birth that indicate that the fetus first acquires the status of human personhood.[2]

The most common signpost is *viability*, that is, the point at which the fetus is able to live on its own outside the womb. Currently, the average fetus is viable at roughly 24 to 26 weeks of gestation, though some fetuses have survived at as early as 20 weeks. Once this point is reached, some argue, the fetus acquires the status of personhood, by virtue of its ability to live on its own, though still heavily dependent on medical technology. The *Roe v. Wade* decision seems to have been premised on this signpost for personhood at the end of the second trimester (the point of viability in 1973).

Viability is not a plausible signpost, because it varies from fetus to fetus, and medical technology is continually pushing viability back to earlier stages of pregnancy. In addition, the concept of viability is a commentary not on the essence of the fetus, but on the ability of medical technology to sustain life outside the womb (a misleading concept since once it leaves the womb the fetus usually trades the natural life-support system of the mother for a temporary, fully artificial one). Viability relates only to the fetus's location and dependency, not to its essence or personhood. There is no inherent connection between the fetus's ability to survive outside the womb and its essential nature as a human being.

Perhaps the next most commonly proposed signpost is *brain development*, or the point at which the brain of the fetus begins to function, at roughly 45 days of pregnancy. The appeal of this signpost is the parallel with the definition of death, which is the cessation of all brain activity. Since the absence of brain activity is what measures death, or the loss of personhood, some argue, it is reasonable to take the beginning of brain activity as an indication that personhood has begun. The problem with the analogy to brain death is that the dead brain is in an irreversible condition, but the fetus only *temporarily* lacks brain function. In addition, the embryo from the point of conception has all the necessary capacities to develop full brain activity. Until around 45 days of gestation those capacities are not yet realized but are latent in the embryo. There are significant differences between the fetus who lacks the capacity for brain activity in normal maturation during the first four to five weeks of pregnancy, and the dead person who lacks both the potentiality and the actuality for any brain activity whatsoever.

A third suggested signpost is *sentience*, or the point at which the fetus is capable of experiencing sensations, particularly pain.[3] As is the case with the other signposts, however, sentience has little inherent connection to the personhood of the fetus, since it confuses the experience of harm with the reality of harm. Simply because the fetus cannot feel pain or otherwise experience harm, it does not follow that it cannot be harmed. If I am paralyzed from the waist down and cannot feel pain in my legs, I am still harmed if someone amputates my leg. In addition, to take sentience as the determinant of personhood, one would also have to admit that the reversibly comatose (the person in a persistent vegetative state as a result of a very serious head injury leaving only the brain stem functioning), the momentarily unconscious, and even the sleeping person are not persons. One might object that these people once did function with sentience and that the loss of sentience is only temporary. But once that objection is made, the objector is admitting that something else besides sentience is determinant of personhood.

A few assert that *birth* is the signpost at which the fetus acquires personhood. But this view is deeply problematic. It seems intuitively obvious that there is no essential difference between the fetus on the day prior to its birth and on the day after its birth. The only difference between the pre-birth and post-birth fetus/newborn is her location. But birth says nothing about what kind of thing the fetus is; it merely offers a commentary on her location and degree of dependence. But just because I change venues, it does not follow that there is any essential change in my nature as a person. Likewise, just because the unborn human substance changes its location, this does not change its essential nature as a fully human being. Even supporters of infanticide recognize that birth is a distinction without an ontological difference, and this is part of the reason for their justification of infanticide.[4]

A final suggested signpost is *implantation*. However, parallel to birth, implantation simply marks a change of location for the fetus. Even if the environment is not suitable for flourishing, it does not follow that location makes an essential difference to what kind of thing the unborn child actually is.

Criteria for Personhood

Given the apparent inadequacies of the above signposts, some suggest that persons must demonstrate certain basic and fundamental functions, often called "criteria for personhood," in order to be considered full persons with the right to life. These include functions such as consciousness/sentience, a developed capacity for reasoning, self-motivated activity, the capacity to communicate, and the ability to have a self-concept.[5] However, the entire project of defining personhood in functional terms fails, since, as argued above, *a thing is what it is, not what it does,* and what it does follows from what it is, not vice versa. Moreover, the absence of expressed functional capacities does not mean that the individual's ultimate ability to express those capacities is absent. Those capacities are simply latent—they have yet to be actualized because the conditions are not yet in place for them to function. Just because capacities are latent, it does not mean that they do not exist, nor does it mean that the person who lacks the expression of them is not a full person, especially if those capacities are latent as a result of the normal maturation of the person. That is, those capacities are latent for a good reason, namely because it is not yet time for them to be actualized in the person's normal process of maturation. Therefore, even if these criteria were among the legitimate identifiers of personhood, every human substance, born and unborn, would qualify as a human person, since a human being is a substance with all the ultimate capacities for fully expressed personhood (though temporarily latent).

The inadequacies of these more functional definitions are clearly evident if we try to practice them consistently. Consider the person under general anesthesia. He is clearly not conscious, has no expressed capacity for reason, is incapable of self-motivated activity, cannot possibly communicate, has no concept of himself, and cannot remember the past or aspire for the future. According to the functionalist view, he is not a full person—but this is absurd. In response, it may be argued that in that state, he or she is a person who is only temporarily dysfunctional. But this claim is not available without appealing to something outside of functional criteria. To argue that the person before anesthesia remains a person while under anesthesia, we must point to what that person is, irrespective of his functional capacities.

Conceding Personhood

Some pro-choice advocates actually concede that the fetus is a person, and yet insist that the pregnant woman's right over her own body outweighs the life of the fetus.[6] She might cite the hypothetical example of the world-renowned violinist who needs a nine-month blood transfusion in order to live. Since you are a perfect match to her blood type, you are drugged and kidnapped. When you wake up, you find yourself hooked up to the violinist and are told that if you unhook yourself, the violinist will die. You then conclude that surely you are not obligated to stay connected to the transfusion machinery for nine months, and that though the fact that the violinist will die if you disconnect is tragic, it is irrelevant to your obligation. She believes that this is analogous to an unwanted pregnancy, that even if the fetus is a person, the mother is not obligated to render nine months' worth of aid, even if failing to do so results in the fetus's death.

Though this analogy to the violinist appears to fit the unwanted pregnancy situation nicely, there are some major differences. First, since the woman was kidnapped and forcibly connected to the transfusion apparatus, this is more analogous to a pregnancy that results from nonconsensual sex, not a pregnancy in which sex is freely engaged. In addition, pregnancy is not comparable to imprisonment, though rarely, some pregnancies require full bed rest and other significant limits on activity. Further, the violinist is a complete stranger. Surely this is not the same thing as a person's child (remember, she has already conceded that the fetus is a person).

Once she has admitted that the fetus is a person, the better analogy is to that of a newborn. Imagine a different hypothetical situation—that you and your spouse have a newborn child, age four months. The baby has not been sleeping more than a couple of hours at any one time, and both of you are exhausted and desperately need a break. So, you decide to take a two-week vacation, just the two of you. But instead of making arrangements for the baby, you prepare enough bottles of formula for two weeks, and you stack two weeks' worth of diapers in the nursery. You then kiss your baby goodbye and leave for two weeks. Upon your return, who do you think would be there to "greet" you? Very angry neighbors, incensed relatives, child protective services, and the police, to arrest you—all of those, and possibly others, would be very interested to see you on your return. The police would likely charge you with child endangerment, and given the high likelihood that your baby died while you were gone, you would also be charged with negligent homicide with callous indifference, if not murder. On what basis would you face those charges? What exactly did you do wrong? You violated the fundamental rights of the baby, not only the right to life, but also the right of the baby to receive what he or she needs from the parents to survive and flourish. We would say that if this is a right of the baby, then *the baby has a claim on the parents* for the resources he or she needs to live and thrive, subject to the ability of the parents to provide them. Of course, if the parents cannot provide at least the minimum of these resources, the state will place the baby into an arrangement where those means are available. If this is true for a newborn, why is it not also true for the fetus? Remember, she has already admitted that the fetus is a person with the right to life. Once she has conceded this, then the mother's right over her own body doesn't trump the baby's right to life. *The baby actually has a claim on the mother's body* for the resources necessary to live and thrive. That's a claim you don't often hear, but one that follows from the concession that the fetus is a person, a sentiment that is growing given the ability of technology to look more clearly at the maturing baby in the womb.

Conclusion

These philosophical reflections on human personhood, as applied to the unborn, are consistent with the biblical teaching that all human beings are image-of-God–bearing persons from conception forward, with continuity of personal identity through time and change. This view—a substance view of a person—is the most plausible way of explaining our common-sense notions of personal identity as well as our concepts of moral responsibility and criminal justice, both of which require a substance view of a person. Our hope in the future is that the erosion of respect for life at both the beginning and ending edges of life can be stopped, and that our culture will recognize that all human beings are members of the human community regardless of their ability or inability to function.

5

Knit Together in a Mother's Womb: The Biology of Prenatal Development

—Tara Sander Lee—

The Heart of Every Human

Have you ever heard the beating heart of an unborn child? It is amazing. The heart is the first organ to form in a developing baby. Heart formation starts approximately 16 days after fertilization.[1] The first heartbeat occurs around day 22, when the woman is only three weeks and one day pregnant.[2] This same heart will beat 54 million times before birth, and over 3.2 billion more times into adulthood, constantly pumping blood through the entire human body for a lifetime.[3]

My own scientific curiosity of the human body started as a young child with my first microscope. Much to my parents' dismay, I started pricking my own finger to look at the blood. The brine shrimp included with the kit paled by comparison to the intricacy and complexity of the human body.

After studying biochemistry as an undergraduate and in graduate school, my research interests led me to Harvard Medical School to study heart and blood vessel formation. The goal was to understand why some children were born with hearts that did not form and function properly. Tiny babies, days after being born, would have to undergo life-saving surgery to repair or replace a part of their heart. Back in the laboratory, I would closely examine the diseased piece of the heart that didn't work correctly. Why didn't the heart develop the way it should? Did the heart cells not grow properly? Did they not mature the way they should? This experience set me on a journey to establish my own research lab and passionately seek to understand causes of pediatric disease.

As I drove to work one day, I heard a haunting broadcast on Christian radio about the number of soldiers who died in all American wars since the Revolution, compared to the number of abortions since the *Roe v. Wade* decision in 1973 to legalize abortion in the United States.[4] Beads were poured into jars and each bead represented 1,000 persons killed. The sound of beads for fallen soldiers was short—a couple seconds. The next set of beads for the millions of babies killed by abortion (now well over 60 million) went on, and on, and on, and on. Tears poured down my face. How could so many babies be killed by abortion? Why would anyone deliberately end the life of a child and intentionally stop his or her beating heart?

Despite the answers to these questions, this is the truth. While countless physicians and scientists work tirelessly to help heal tiny human hearts with medical advancements, abortion clinics nationwide use high-powered suction machines and toxic chemicals to terminate the beating hearts and lives of millions of babies. The heartrending contradiction is overwhelming.

Abortion is even harder to understand when you desire to have a biological child of your own. My husband and I struggled for years with infertility and suffered pregnancy losses. An *in vitro* fertilization procedure produced three fertilized embryos, but resulted in no pregnancy, and even caused a life-threatening complication requiring hospitalization. We experienced two first-trimester miscarriages from natural pregnancy—one was twins. Sacred reminders that every human being—no matter how young, no matter how they were created, and no matter how many days they lived, whether inside or outside the womb—is precious.

The Preborn as Persons

Sadly, so many innocent babies have been killed by abortion because they are not regarded as persons. Women facing an unplanned pregnancy are told a lie, that the child growing inside of them is not a real human being, despite countless biology and embryology textbooks, scientists, and medical professionals saying otherwise. Planned Parenthood, the world's largest abortion provider, dehumanizes the preborn at every turn. The word "baby" is never mentioned during pregnancy. Instead, "pregnancy tissue," and other such lifeless terms are used to describe the developing baby.[5] Another organization tells women to "flush everything down the toilet" and "throw them away" when completing a chemical abortion at home.[6] Pregnancy is described as a never-ending series of unpleasant symptoms that would terrify any mother, listing them as "discomforts," month by month, that "usually get worse" and are "troublesome." The joy to be experienced in pregnancy is concealed. The humanity of the child is abandoned. Science is ignored.

Webster's dictionary defines a "person" as a "human being" or "individual," separate and distinct from another.[7] Personhood is not governed by age, stage of development, level of dependency on another, abilities, or capacity to do certain things. If that were so, then newborn babies, the disabled, elderly, those suffering with debilitating disease, and anyone who is not fully "functional" or is dependent on another, would not be considered a person. How we function does not make us more or less of a person. Instead, personhood can be explained by science and biology, the natural world, and what defines us as human beings.

How do we share the truth that the preborn are human beings from the very beginning, with intrinsic value and worth? Every child in the womb is a precious, unique life, handcrafted by God in His own image—a person in every sense of the word, deserving of respect, dignity, and life. How do we firmly yet graciously arm individuals with scientific facts for defending life, when so many oppose and choose to ignore the science?

Human Life Begins at Conception

Centuries of scientific discovery and technological advancement have provided indisputable proof that from the moment of conception, when the sperm fertilizes the egg, there is the creation of a new, totally distinct, integrated organism—a human being (a person), biologically distinct from all other life forms on this planet. The dynamics of fertilization and human development are well-established. In fact, the very first stage of human development is called Carnegie Stage 1a, marked by the moment of fertilization.[8] The Carnegie

Stages of Human Development were first established in 1942, have since been expanded, and remain the standard used by *all* biologists to describe the first eight weeks of human life.[9]

At the moment of fertilization, key steps are initiated that begin development of a new human organism. Each cell contains all of the fundamental molecules it needs to grow, mature, and function, from the very beginning, and for the rest of his or her life.[10] DNA is one of these most basic, fundamental molecules. DNA is in all living things and is passed on from generation to generation, fashioning distinctive characteristics and distinct traits to each next living thing. Human gametes (the sperm and egg) each contain 23 chromosomes, half the number of chromosomes needed to be a human organism. The union of the male and female DNA during fertilization restores the number of 46 chromosomes needed to create a human being with a complete set of unchangeable DNA for that individual's entire life.

In Psalm 139, King David wrote that our frame was not hidden from God when made in the secret place and knit together in our mother's womb.[11] Centuries after this psalm was written, scientists Watson and Crick proposed the structure of DNA—the blueprint of life—in their seminal 1953 *Nature* paper. They described DNA as "two ribbons" of genetic material woven together.[12] In the same way that letters of the alphabet combine to create an unlimited number of unique words for communicating, so it is with DNA. The nucleotide "letters" (A, C, G, T) of DNA join together like beads on a string and combine in different ways to create various messages (or genes) for specific functions within the cell.

Every living thing has its own unique genome (or complete DNA code), based on the same four nucleotides, A-C-G-T. For example, the genome of a fly is different from a worm, which is different from a mouse and a monkey. Comparing the genomes of various species has revealed that *Homo sapiens* have a genome that is distinctly human and distinguishable from all other animals and plants. For example, human beings have unique DNA, not found in any other animals, that appears to be responsible for why humans have bigger and more complex brains compared to other species.[13]

God designed each person to be unique and magnificent from the moment of conception. The earliest human embryo starts as a single cell, grows to nearly one billion cells by the end of the eighth embryonic week, and will become a fully developed adult containing 30 to 40 trillion cells.[14] The complete genome for each human being is present at conception in the earliest single-cell embryo. There are approximately three billion base pairs of DNA sequence in each human diploid cell;[15] "diploid" refers to a cell that contains two complete sets of chromosomes, i.e., one from each parent. No two humans ever have been or will be genetically the same. Even in the case of identical twins, they don't share identical fingerprints, and most have small differences in DNA. When estimating the number of different types of people that can be created, it has been determined that any male and female couple can produce 8,388,608 offspring that are each genetically unique.[16] The probability of there being two identical children from any two parents in the population is 6.27 billion to one.[17] If all the DNA in any adult human body is unraveled like a string, it would exceed 63 billion miles in length, which is comparable to 340 round trips from the earth to the sun and back![18]

Even leading biologists confirm that life begins at conception. Embryologists Ronan O'Rahilly and Fabiola Müller noted that while life is a continuous process, fertilization is "a critical landmark" at which "a new, genetically distinct human organism is formed," with further observation that, "Just as prenatal age begins at fertilization, postnatal age begins at birth."[19] Non-scientists also acknowledge that human life begins at conception. Pro-choice, atheist philosopher Peter Singer has stated, "There is no doubt that from the first moments of its existence, an embryo conceived from human sperm and eggs is a human being."[20] And Margaret Sanger, the founder of Planned Parenthood, stated that, "no new life begins unless there is conception."[21]

A more recent 2019 research study from the University of Chicago quantified the number of biologists who confirm that life begins at fertilization. Results from the study verified that of the 5,577 biologists surveyed, 96 percent affirmed that a human life begins at fertilization.[22] Responses were based on scientific fact, regardless of differing views on abortion and politics.[23] In fact, the majority of the sample identified as liberal (89%), pro-choice (85%), nonreligious (63%) and Democrats (92%). The conclusion from this study is simple—the vast majority of biologists agree that all human life begins at the moment of conception, because it is scientifically true and based on validated, objective, biological investigation.

Stages of Human Development

Human development is a growth continuum, marked by several key stages that occur within the first eight weeks of human embryonic development (e.g., Carnegie stages 1–23).[24] The developing human baby is called an embryo from the time of fertilization until the end of the eighth week of gestation. From the beginning of the ninth week of gestation until birth, the baby is called a fetus. These definitional terms and time frames have been recognized by leading scientists and scientific organizations for decades.

There are two main methods for dating a pregnancy and the age of the preborn. Most obstetricians use an older system, measured from the first day of the woman's last menstrual period (LMP) to the current date. This method of dating is also known as gestational age or ovulation age. Embryologists often date pregnancy from the start of conception, also known as "post-fertilization" date. The length of pregnancy is 38 weeks, from time of fertilization (or conception) until birth, or 40 weeks gestational age. For the purposes of this essay, the age of the preborn is based on post-fertilization dates.

Key pathways have been identified that reveal the many complex and intricate molecular, cellular, and structural factors and interactions that contribute to formation of a human being. These dynamics begin at fertilization, continue through embryo and fetal development, and last for a lifetime. The most significant milestones of human development occur during the eight weeks after fertilization. It is during this embryonic period when the body parts and organ systems become visible and start to function. For example, it has been estimated that there are 4,500 body parts in adults, and 4,000 of these structures are formed within the first eight weeks of human development.[25] This scientific fact alone reveals the tremendous level of masterwork involved in the making of every human life, especially at the very beginning. Numerous biological discoveries and advancements in fetal imaging have revealed many other fascinating scientific facts. We know when the heart starts beating, when fingerprints are formed, when hairs on the head develop, when the fetus feels pain, yawns, hiccups, responds to sound and light, sleeps, and possibly even dreams—all before birth. Countless scientific resources, academic research articles, and embryology textbooks have recorded these key events. A brief summary is provided as evidence below, to deepen your understanding and knowledge of how every human life—every person—is formed inside the womb and is "fearfully and wonderfully made" (Ps. 139:14).

Human Embryonic Development[26]

After conception, a new human organism is a one-cell embryo, called a *zygote*. The embryo is about 100 microns in size, which is smaller than a speck of sand. The sex of the embryo is determined genetically at fertilization by the pair of sex chromosomes (XX–female; XY–male). The human embryo undergoes rapid growth within the first week, through a process of repeated cell division called cleavage. After the first cell division, the one-cell embryo will become two cells. More divisions result in four cells, then eight cells, and finally at a 16-cell stage, the embryo is a *morula*. The developing embryo continues to grow and move through the fallopian tube. The embryo enters the uterus as an early *blastocyst,* which contains an inner cell mass consisting of about 200 cells, called embryonic stem cells. These stem cells will eventually give rise to all the tissues and organs of the human body, including the heart, lung, brain, etc. The human embryo has a specialized outer layer called the *trophoblast,* which enables the attachment and implantation of the embryo into the endometrium (the lining of the womb). The embryo's cells begin to create a hormone called human chorionic gonadotropin (hCG), the hormone detected by pregnancy tests.

Implantation is completed by the second week. The embryo is now in a permanent home within his or her mother and will stay there until fully developed and ready for birth. The mother's body undergoes dramatic changes to provide nourishment and nutrients to her child. The placenta begins to form and, once fully developed, will serve as an important barrier and interface, protecting the baby from many infections and delivering oxygen and nutrients to the developing child.[27]

By the third week, the human body plan is forming. The embryo has three distinct layers (ectoderm, mesoderm, and endoderm), which will give rise to all of the tissues and organ systems. The ectoderm layer forms skin, the central nervous system, hair, nails, and many other structures. The endoderm layer forms the lining of the respiratory system, the gut and its derivatives. And the mesoderm layer forms the blood vessels, bone, connective tissue, and other supportive structures. The brain is also dividing into its primary sections: the forebrain, midbrain, and hindbrain.

The first blood cells appear in the yolk sac, blood vessels start to form throughout the embryo, as the tubular heart emerges. Once the growing heart folds in upon itself, separate chambers begin to develop. And at 22 days after fertilization, the baby's heart beats for the first time. By the time most women determine they are pregnant, the heart will have already started to form into a fully functioning organ. Within about another week, the heart is beating rhythmically. At 3 to 4 weeks, the human body plan emerges and the brain, spinal cord, and heart alongside the yolk sac can easily be identified.

During weeks 4 and 5, the limb buds (upper and lower) start to appear, which will become flattened to form the hand- and footplates. The brain continues to grow, the eyes and liver are developing, and permanent kidneys appear. The yolk sac contains early reproductive cells called primordial germ cells, which begin migrating to the developing gonads (reproductive organs), adjacent to the kidneys.

During weeks 5 and 6, eye pigment and the retina start forming. Nerves enter the upper limb buds and digital rays begin to form the bones of the thumb and fingers in each hand. White blood cells (called lymphocytes) are produced by the liver as the immune system develops. The heart and lungs move deeper into the chest. Pain receptors start to develop, first around the mouth, and will cover the body by 18 weeks.

During weeks 6 and 7, the cerebral hemispheres are growing

faster than other regions of the human body. The embryo starts to make spontaneous and reflexive movements, thus promoting neuromuscular development. Brainwaves in the developing human brain can be detected as early as 6 weeks, 2 days after fertilization. The external ear is beginning to take shape. Blood cell formation is underway in the liver, where lymphocytes are now present. The immune system is developing and white blood cells are produced. Elbows may be identifiable and the fingers are beginning to separate.

During weeks 7 and 8, hiccups have been observed. Taste buds start to appear. Leg movements can be seen along with startle response. The hands and feet of the baby can move together. Human brain activity can be recorded. In fact, the human brain will continue to develop and mature even after birth and well into the person's twenties. If the embryo is touched, there may be squinting, jaw movement, grasping motions, or toe pointing. Kidneys produce urine. The skin becomes multilayered and is less transparent. Eyebrows start to appear. Eyelids are forming. The gonads start acquiring male and female morphological characteristics (i.e., ovaries in females, testes produce testosterone in males).

During weeks 8 and 9, the baby can suck her thumb, swallow amniotic fluid, grasp an object, move the head, move the tongue, sigh, and stretch. The baby has nerve receptors in the face, hands, and feet allowing him or her to sense and respond to light touch. Cells from the embryo are migrating into the mother's blood and circulate through her bloodstream.[28] Scientists can detect the baby's DNA in the mother's blood, before birth, and screen for genetic mutations. The identification of a DNA mutation is sometimes used as justification to abort the baby. In fact, this modern form of eugenics is causing the rapid decline of certain populations, particularly persons who carry an extra chromosome 21 (Trisomy 21) causing Down syndrome.

Human Fetal Development

From the beginning of the ninth week of gestation until birth, the baby is called a fetus. During weeks 9 and 10, the vocal cords are starting to develop. External genitals start to distinguish male and female. The fetus can yawn. Fingernails and toenails are forming. The person's unique fingerprints are starting to develop. During weeks 10 and 11, the nose and lips are completely formed. Male and female are now distinguishable by genitalia. During weeks 11 and 12, bowel movements begin. The baby touches his or her mouth regularly. Twelve weeks marks the end of the first trimester of pregnancy.

During the second trimester (12 to 25 weeks), the fetus undergoes significant additional development. The tiny child can swallow, scrunch hands into little fists, touch their face, and scratch their head. The baby's fingers and toes are also complete with nails. At 13 weeks, the fetal heart pumps about 26 quarts of blood per day, and this number will continue to increase, pumping about 2,000 quarts of blood per day at birth! Fingerprints are fully developed by 14 weeks. Between weeks 14 to 18, pregnant women can feel the baby kicking, known as "quickening." Pain receptors completely cover the body by 18 weeks, and brain structures are mature enough to process pain. At 18 weeks, the baby's ears can hear music and recognize their mother's voice. By 20 weeks, the cochlea has reached adult size. Hair grows on the scalp. By 24 weeks, eyelids reopen and the fetus can blink. The baby will react to loud noises. And there is significant rapid brain growth.

Ultrasound screening during the second trimester (usually around 20 weeks) can detect structural anomalies. Birth defects are the leading cause of infant mortality and morbidity, affecting approximately one in every 33 live births (about 3 percent) in the

United States each year and accounting for 20 percent of all infant deaths.[29] By 21 to 22 weeks, the lungs gain some ability to function on their own. As early as 20 weeks, it is possible for babies to be born and survive outside the womb with medical intervention. Between weeks 14 to 24 (on average), doctors can treat preborn babies with life-saving therapies, and repair significant defects for certain diseases—such as twin-to-twin transfusion syndrome, a life-threatening condition in which the blood flows unequally between twins who share a placenta, and spina bifida, a neural tube disorder causing the spine to not develop properly.[30] Pain medication is routinely administered as standard medical practice during fetal surgery procedures, because preborn persons feel pain. At 22 to 23 weeks, a fetus will respond to pain with the same behaviors as older babies: scrunching up the eyes, opening the mouth, clenching hands, withdrawing the limbs.[31]

During the third trimester (26 to 38 weeks), the fetus undergoes tremendous growth. By 26 weeks, eyes produce tears. By 27 weeks, pupils respond to light. The baby can be seen making altered facial expressions and performing somersaults! By 28 weeks, the fetus can distinguish between high and low pitch sounds. By 30 weeks, breathing patterns are more common. True alveoli develop in lungs by 32 weeks and continue to develop until eight years after birth. The baby's hands can make a firm grasp. At 38 weeks, the fetus initiates labor and there is childbirth.

There are so many more events that occur during the various stages of human development, but it is not possible to describe them all in this essay. The ones mentioned here are small highlights of the countless miraculous events happening inside the womb.

Conclusion

My husband and I finally did become pregnant. We saw our son's heartbeat, his legs kick, and facial expressions—all before birth. My son is the same person now as he was when he was first conceived. Inside the womb, he was just a smaller snapshot of the larger person he would later become outside the womb. The same blue eyes that developed inside me are the same blue eyes that look back at me now with amazement when I tell him he used to be smaller than a speck of sand. There is awe and humility in every created life. Every human being developing in the womb is a person, and ending their life, at any stage of development, interrupts a divine masterplan. As the Lord told the prophet Jeremiah, "Before I formed you in the womb, I knew you" (Jer. 1:5 NIV).

These truths are very real for me. I have been profoundly impacted by two women who faced an unplanned pregnancy and, despite the option to abort, chose life. Each of these women was carrying a baby boy and, after birth, selflessly gave up their child in order to give them a home that they could not provide. Because of these courageous women, I have two adopted brothers. My mother became pregnant as a teenager, so my older half-brother was adopted *out* to another family before I was born. Almost forty years later, he searched for his biological mother, my mother, and we have been reunited as a family ever since. On the other hand, my younger brother was adopted *into* our family as a newborn when I was eight years old.

I may not know my two brothers in the same way, but I do know they were both meant to *be*. These are real people—living and breathing persons—who laugh, love, cry, and feel pain. They are each unique and one of a kind. The same person who was conceived in the womb is the same person who was born, had a first birthday, became an adult, got married, and had beautiful children of their own. A whole new generation is born and in existence because they live, because their birth mothers chose to give them *life*. Just think about all the thousands of lives, including mine, that would never have been touched had they not been born.

The state of Louisiana recognizes that every human being, from the moment of conception, is a "*person*," with equal rights deserving of protection.[32] Under Louisiana Health Law, "a viable *in vitro* fertilized human ovum is a juridical person," with legal status, "which shall not be intentionally destroyed by any natural or other juridical person or through the actions of any other such person." Such protections are important for the millions of embryos generated by *in vitro* fertilization procedures that are considered to be "extras" and are not implanted into a woman for pregnancy. These "leftover" embryos are often discarded or donated to research, where they are eventually destroyed for science experiments (embryonic stem cell research, heritable genome editing, cloning, etc.). Human embryos can also be frozen and stored indefinitely.

But some couples choose a life-saving option for these cherished embryos. They donate their "extra" embryos to another family for adoption (also known as "snowflake babies"). Since the 1990s, over 7,000 babies have been born to families through embryo adoption.[33] The National Embryo Donation Center in Knoxville, Tennessee, was recently the first embryo adoption program in the world to mark a 1,000-birth milestone, with the birth of a little girl, named Emmie Sue.[34] Embryo adoption is a wonderful way to help families that are struggling with infertility, while honoring the dignity and life of each human embryo. As one physician notes, "Every single one of those 1000 babies has their own unique story."[35]

Science has unveiled how every baby developing in the womb does *indeed* have their own "unique story" to tell. The scientific facts and testimonies presented in this essay should embolden you to stand and bear witness to the truth. Every preborn child is a person, a human being, and a complete member of the human species—from conception, through all stages of embryo and fetal development, until birth. It is essential that we defend the sanctity of every human life, created by God in His own image, and serve as a voice for the most vulnerable and defenseless among us, at a time when they most desperately need it.

6

Equal Protection for the Preborn: A Case for Prenatal Personhood according to the Fourteenth Amendment

—Joshua J. Craddock—

The 1973 Supreme Court decision *Roe v. Wade* required states to allow abortion.[1] The seven men forming the majority said the right to privacy includes a woman's decision to end the life of her preborn child, effectively through all nine months of pregnancy. During initial arguments for *Roe,* Texas argued that "the fetus is a 'person' within the language and meaning of the Fourteenth Amendment."[2] The Supreme Court rejected that conclusion and ruled "that the word 'person,' as used in the Fourteenth Amendment, does not include the unborn."[3]

Even legal scholars who agree in principle with the outcome of *Roe* have roundly criticized the Court's blanket approach to creating a federally protected right to abortion.[4] When *Roe* determined that states could not protect preborn humans as persons, "the Court effectively decided that the Constitution requires their exclusion."[5] Nevertheless, the Justice who wrote the *Roe v. Wade* opinion, Harry Blackmun, made an important admission. He wrote: If prenatal "personhood is established," the case for abortion "collapses, for the fetus' right to life would then be guaranteed specifically by the [Fourteenth] Amendment."[6]

The Fourteenth Amendment was ratified in 1868, after the Civil War, to ensure that no human being would be denied fundamental rights guaranteed by the Constitution. The Amendment says:

> No State shall . . . deprive any person of life, liberty, or property, without due process of law; nor deny to any person within its jurisdiction the equal protection of the laws.[7]

Other essays in this volume seek to demonstrate the personhood of the preborn by way of other academic disciplines. In this essay we will take up Justice Blackmun's challenge from a decidedly legal angle, namely by examining whether the preborn are implicated in the Fourteenth Amendment by virtue of the language of the Amendment itself. Are unborn children "persons" within the original public meaning of the Fourteenth Amendment?

From one perspective, the story of our Constitution—and the Fourteenth Amendment in particular—has been the story of extending the protection of fundamental legal rights to more and more classes of persons, including African Americans, Native Americans, women, non-citizen aliens, the developmentally disabled, and illegitimate children. In every case, the affirmation of constitutional guarantees for these classes of persons was based on their mere status as human beings within the Constitution's juridical reach. Even when the parameters of equal protection and due process are tailored to their subjects, such as the more circumscribed rights held by children and non-citizens, the core of those guarantees are recognized in some way for all members of the human family within the borders of the United States—except for our youngest members. Indeed, even the Universal Declaration of Human Rights declares that "everyone has the right to recognition everywhere as a person before the law."[8]

Another perspective considers the original meaning of the Fourteenth Amendment and looks to the meaning of the text at the time it was written and ratified. Using this interpretive method, one might look to dictionaries of legal and common usage, the context of the common-law tradition, and the original expectations of those who drafted the Amendment as evidence of its meaning. Using this methodology, it is reasonable to conclude that the Fourteenth Amendment guarantees unborn children due process of law and the equal protection of the laws.

The structure of this argument is simple.[9] The Fourteenth Amendment's use of the word "person" guarantees due process and equal protection to all members of the human species. The preborn are members of the human species from the moment of fertilization.[10] Therefore, the Amendment protects the preborn. If one concedes the minor premise (that preborn humans are members of the human species), all that must be demonstrated is that the term "person," *in its original public meaning at the time of the Fourteenth Amendment's adoption*, applied to all members of the human species.

The minor premise need not be lingered upon here. Nevertheless, we should observe that whether states historically believed the preborn were members of the human species is not dispositive, so long as they believed all human beings were entitled to protection under the Fourteenth Amendment. Just as "freedom of speech" protects movies and internet communication under the original meaning—even though those technologies were not invented at the time of the First Amendment's adoption—"person" protects every member of the human species, regardless of whether individuals were recognized as members of the human family at the time of the Fourteenth Amendment's adoption.[11]

The major premise may be defended with three lines of evidence. First, textual analysis, such as dictionary definitions from the period; second, common-law precedent and state practice; and third, the Amendment's anticipated legal application.

Textual Inferences and Dictionary Usage

According to dictionaries of common and legal usage at the time of the Fourteenth Amendment's adoption, the term "person" was largely interchangeable with "human being" or "man."[12] The 1864 edition of Noah Webster's *American Dictionary of the English Language* defined the term "person" as relating "especially [to] a living human being; a man, woman, or child; an individual of the human race."[13] The entry for "human" includes all those belonging to "the race of man."[14] No dictionary of the era referenced birth or the status of being born in its definition of "person," "man," or "human being."[15]

In legal usage, the term "person" had expansive scope. In his discourse on "The Rights of Persons," eighteenth-century legal scholar William Blackstone wrote that "natural persons are such as the God of nature formed us."[16] Blackstone made no distinction between the *biological* fact of humanity and the *legal* status of personhood.[17] He considered all members of the human species to be legal persons.

Blackstone declared that "life is . . . a right inherent by nature in every individual; and it begins in contemplation of law as soon as an infant is able to stir in the mother's womb."[18] Mention of the preborn child's stirring was intended to protect prenatal life as soon as it could be discerned, not to exclude human life from protection prior to that point. For Blackstone, if human life existed, legal personhood existed also.[19]

Instead of exploring the term's original meaning and historical usage, the *Roe* Court used an intratextual methodology to ply the meaning of "person."[20] Of course, it is difficult to prove what a term *cannot* mean through negative inferences alone.[21] Yet it was through this method that Justice Blackmun concluded "person" cannot include the preborn.[22]

For instance, consider the first sentence of the Amendment: "All persons born or naturalized in the United States, and subject to the jurisdiction thereof, are citizens of the United States."[23] It does not define the scope of the class "persons."[24] Rather, the phrases "born or naturalized" and "subject to the jurisdiction thereof" serve to narrow the broader class of *persons* to define its subset, *citizens.*[25]

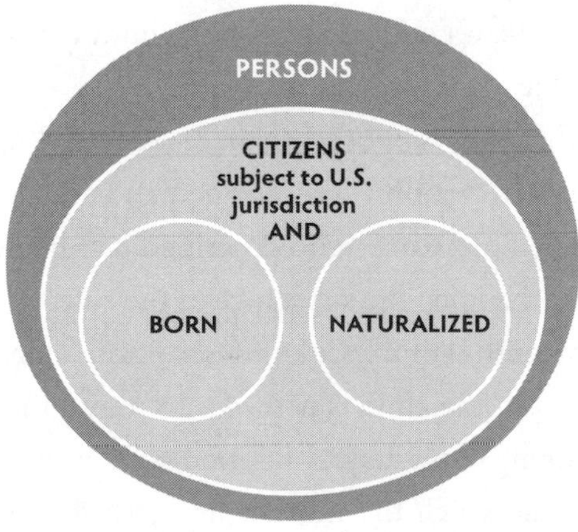

Other constitutional clauses serve to narrow the broader class of "persons" for other purposes, such as electoral apportionment or eligibility for federal office. But none can be interpreted to limit the meaning of "person" only to post-natal application. Textual analysis and examination of dictionary usage actually supports the conclusion that preborn human beings are included within the sweep of the Fourteenth Amendment's protection.

Common Law Precedent and State Practice

By the time of the Fourteenth Amendment's adoption, nearly every state prohibited abortion in its criminal code,[26] and most of those statutes were classified as "offenses against the person."[27] Indeed, in twenty-three states and six territories, laws referred to the preborn individual as a "child."[28] Is it reasonable to presume that state legislatures would have used this terminology unless they believed the child in utero to be a "person"?[29]

The adoption of strict anti-abortion measures in the mid-nineteenth century was the natural development of a long common-law history proscribing abortion. Beginning in the mid-thirteenth century, the common law codified abortion as homicide as soon as the child came to life—that is, as soon as the child was "formed and animated."[30] This was supposed to have occurred approximately forty days after fertilization.[31] The "formed and animated" standard was later cited by Lord Coke, who described it as being "quick with childe" without changing the substance of the rule.[32]

In the eighteenth century, Coke's description "quick with childe" (the point at which the child is first *able* to move, then considered to be the beginning of existence) became equivocal with "quickening" (the point at which the mother first *feels* fetal movement).[33]

As explained above, the quickening rule was intended to protect prenatal life as soon as it could be discerned, not to exclude human life from protection prior to that point. The *Roe* Court made much of the quickening rule in its rush to dismiss the personhood of the preborn,[34] but failed to see that the rule was merely a tool of criminal law, not a statement about the value of life prior to perceptible movement in the womb.

The "quickening" distinction survived in common law until emergent medical science discovered "that human life began at fertilization,"[35] allowing medical examiners to prove prenatal life and cause of death due to abortion with greater certainty. After this discovery in the early nineteenth century, British courts instructed jurors that "quick with child" (which had earlier meant "formed and animated") now meant "from the moment of conception."[36] When determining whether to grant temporary reprieve from execution for a pregnant woman, for example, *Regina v. Wycherley* reinterpreted common law to reflect new scientific fact in 1838.[37]

This revision of the common law to conform to this basic principle—that human life, where it exists, must be protected—informed the meaning of the term "person" in the United States at the time of the Fourteenth Amendment's adoption. Thomas Percival's influential and widely circulated nineteenth century work *Medical Ethics* declared, "To extinguish the first spark of life is a crime of the same nature, both against our Maker and society, as to destroy an infant, a child, or a man."[38] The American Medical Association's 1859 report on abortion considered the human being in utero a person, and it called for protection of the "independent and actual existence of the child before birth, as a living being."[39] It decried the "unnecessary and unjustifiable destruction of human life" both before and after quickening, and they urged state legislatures to reform their abortion statutes.[40] The Medical Society of New York in 1867 "condemned abortion at every stage of gestation, as 'murder.'"[41]

In the mid-nineteenth century, American courts began to discard the obsolete "quickening" standard in favor of protecting the unborn from the time of fertilization.[42] The Pennsylvania Supreme Court's ruling in 1850 is indicative of the national mood regarding abortion in that era. It wrote, "the moment the womb is instinct with embryo life, and gestation has begun, the crime may be perpetrated. . . . There was therefore a crime at common law."[43] The Supreme Judicial Court of Maine similarly upheld a statute repudiating the quickening standard in its 1851 *Smith v. State* decision.[44]

Meanwhile, state legislatures took action to prohibit abortion from the time of fertilization. At the end of 1849, eighteen of the thirty states had legally proscribed abortion.[45] By the end of 1864, that number grew to twenty-seven of the thirty-six states. When the Fourteenth Amendment was adopted in 1868, the states widely recognized children in utero as persons: at the close of that year, it was thirty out of thirty-seven, plus six territories.[46] Of those thirty states in 1868, twenty-seven punished abortion irrespective of quickening and twenty applied the same punishment before and after quickening.[47] Twenty-three states and six territories referred to the fetus as a "child" in their statutes proscribing abortion.[48] At least twenty-eight jurisdictions labeled abortion as an "offense against the person" or an equivalent criminal classification.[49] Although minor policy-driven differences existed among states in the treatment of abortion at common law, a general consensus treated preborn human beings as "persons."

Nine of the ratifying states explicitly treated the preborn as equal persons to their pregnant mothers by providing the same range of punishment for killing either during the commission of an abortion.[50] Furthermore, ten states (nine of which had ratified the Fourteenth Amendment) considered abortion to be either manslaughter, assault with intent to murder, or murder.[51] New York joined them in 1869, and the number grew to seventeen jurisdictions in the period shortly after the adoption of the Fourteenth Amendment.[52] A significant number of states also considered actions that, while not intended to cause abortion, caused the death of a child in utero to be manslaughter.[53]

Several states left clear documentary evidence about their legislative purposes, which sheds light on how lawmakers viewed the relationship between these statutes and the Fourteenth Amendment. Take Ohio, for example. After ratifying the Fourteenth Amendment in January 1867, the Ohio legislature took up a bill to amend their 1834 anti-abortion statute.[54] The committee that reviewed the bill was composed of several senators who had voted for ratification of the amendment.[55]

Their Senate report explained the purposes of the statute, observing "the alarming and increasing frequency" of abortion by "a class of quacks who make child-murder a trade."[56] Pointing out that "physicians have now arrived at the unanimous opinion that the foetus in utero is alive from the very moment of conception," the committee repudiated the "'ridiculous distinction' in the punishment of abortion before and after quickening."[57] They asserted that "no opinion could be more erroneous" than to think "that to destroy the embryo before that period [of quickening] is not child-murder."[58] They concluded their report: "Let it be proclaimed to the world, and let it be impressed upon the conscience of every woman in the land 'that the willful killing of a human being, at any stage of its existence, is murder.'"[59] The bill passed both houses of the Ohio legislature by April 1867.[60]

Other state legislatures that ratified the Fourteenth Amendment were of the same opinion.[61] This may be inferred from the language these legislatures used, that these legislatures enacted anti-abortion statutes at the request of state medical societies (which had asserted the personhood of the unborn as the justification for new anti-abortion measures), and that these legislatures did not view their proscriptions of abortion as inconsistent with the Amendment.[62]

At the time of the Fourteenth Amendment, nearly all of the states understood "person" to include prenatal life. The inclusive meaning of "person" in 1860s state law should thus persuasively inform an originalist understanding of the Amendment.

Anticipated Legal Application

The legislatures that in short sequence adopted anti-abortion statutes and ratified the Fourteenth Amendment saw no conflict between their actions to defend prenatal life and their Fourteenth Amendment obligations.[63] Indeed, they may have even viewed such legislation as *required* by the Amendment. The framers of the Amendment certainly thought it required protection of every human being.

The framers expected the Fourteenth Amendment to protect every member of the human species. The Amendment was carefully worded to "bring within the aegis of the due process and equal protection clauses every member of the human race, regardless of age, imperfection or condition of unwantedness."[64] Senator Jacob Howard, who sponsored the Amendment in the Senate, declared the Amendment's purpose to "disable a State from depriving not merely a citizen of the United States, but any person, whoever he may be, of life, liberty, or property without due process of law."[65] Even the lowest and "most despised of the [human] race" were guaranteed the equal protection.[66] Representative Thaddeus Stevens called the Amendment "a superstructure of perfect equality of every human being before the law; of impartial protection to every one in whose breast God had placed an immortal soul."[67] Representative James Brown simply put it: "Does the term 'person' carry with it anything further than a simple allusion to the existence of the individual?"[68]

The primary framer of the Fourteenth Amendment, Representative John Bingham, intended it to ensure that "no state in the Union should deny to any human being . . . the equal protection of the laws."[69] He described the Amendment as a remedy to the denial of basic human rights, to ensure no state would, "in its madness or its folly refuse to the gentleman, or *his children or to me or to mine,* any of the rights which pertain to American citizenship or to common humanity."[70]

Though Bingham never addressed the issue of abortion, the general consensus of 1868 was that prenatal life was human and therefore included within common humanity. The Amendment cannot therefore be legitimately interpreted "to exclude a group of individuals who were regarded as human beings at the time the fourteenth amendment was written."[71]

Certainly the Amendment's framers did not promote an understanding of "legal personhood" separate from biological humanity.[72] Indeed, they would have looked to the long-established precedent of *United States v. Palmer,* in which Chief Justice Marshall acknowledged that the terms "person or persons" were broad enough to include "every human being" and "the whole human race."[73] The authors of the amendment designed it to protect all biological human beings, regardless of their origin or circumstance. As Justice Hugo Black later put it: "the history of the [Fourteenth] amendment proves that the people were told that its purpose was to protect weak and helpless human beings."[74]

Given the original public meaning of the term "person," the contemporaneous anti-abortion statutes purposed to protect prenatal life, and the public explanations given by the framers of the Fourteenth Amendment as to the Amendment's scope of meaning, the evidence indicates the framers had no intention to exclude the unborn from the Amendment's protection. The Fourteenth Amendment was to be a new birth of freedom for *all* human beings.

Conclusion

Roe v. Wade and its progeny are constitutionally unsound. Unborn children are constitutionally entitled to due process and the equal protection of the laws. The Fourteenth Amendment, properly interpreted, prohibits any state from allowing abortion, and every officer who swears an oath to uphold the Constitution has a duty to ensure those rights are protected.

What would happen if a state permitted abortion? If prenatal life is to be protected under the Fourteenth Amendment, the federal government must intervene in states that do not guarantee equal protection and due process to preborn human beings. Should a state refuse to protect prenatal life, it would be a violation of equal protection as understood in the *Civil Rights Cases*[75] and later reiterated in *Bell v. Maryland*:

> "Denying includes inaction as well as action. And denying the equal protection of the laws includes the omission to protect, as well as the omission to pass laws for protection." These views are fully consonant with this Court's

> recognition that state conduct which might be described as "inaction" can nevertheless constitute responsible "state action" within the meaning of the Fourteenth Amendment.[76]

Failing to prosecute the intentional killing of unborn persons while prosecuting the homicide of members of other classes of persons is an equal protection violation.[77] *Reitman v. Mulkey* determined that statutes permissive of individual discriminatory actions can constitute state action violating the Equal Protection Clause.[78] This reasoning has been relied upon by inferior court decisions requiring life-saving blood transfusions for fetuses, even against their parents' religious objections.[79] In one such case, the justices were unanimously "satisfied that the unborn child is entitled to the law's protection" from inaction that would deprive her of life.[80] Applying the same principle, a state's consistent and systematic failure to act warrants federal intervention. Given the broad agreement among the states which held that unborn children are "persons under criminal, tort, and property law, the text of the Equal Protection Clause of the Fourteenth Amendment compels federal protection of unborn persons."[81]

The Supreme Court's abortion jurisprudence demonstrates the need to reexamine the Court's role as the final arbiter of constitutional meaning and fundamental rights. Each branch and level of government has a role to play. Congress should act under Section 5 of the Fourteenth Amendment to "enforce, by appropriate legislation," the Constitution's protections for unborn persons.[82] The Executive should follow President Lincoln's example and assert his departmental authority to interpret and uphold the Constitution, fulfilling his constitutional duty to "take Care that the Laws be faithfully executed."[83] This may and should include a rejection of the judicial supremacy implicit in the notion that *Roe v. Wade* is "the law of the land." After all, the President swears an oath to preserve the *Constitution*, not every pronouncement of the Supreme Court.

States retain the primary duty to protect the inalienable rights of all human beings within their jurisdictions, the foremost of which is the right to life. States have a responsibility to exercise their police powers (their powers to promote public health, safety, and morals) to prohibit abortion. State governors and legislators must do everything in their power to uphold the Constitution on this point.

Ultimately, it is the people's responsibility to dismantle the separate and unequal caste system that discriminates against unborn human beings, with their voices and their votes. Only they can bring science and law into harmony in a manner consistent with the Constitution. And only they can ensure that the equal protection of the laws is guaranteed to *all* persons.

CLAIM 3

My Body, My Choice

7

Whose Body? The Illusion of Autonomy

—D. Joy Riley—

"Nan" and I became friends in graduate school. She invited me to her apartment for dinner one evening. I was surprised to see something beyond the usual graduate student fare. Sometime during the meal, she told me that it was a special day: the tenth anniversary of the day her child had been aborted. I expressed condolences but did not know what else to say to my friend who seemed conflicted as she marked this day. I mostly listened.

Years later, I have no small number of post-abortive women among my friends. Most are mothers of other, living children, but a few are not. Each has her own story, yet most report some resemblance to the experience described by "Jane Doe" (Linda Bird Francke) in her *New York Times* essay, "There Just Wasn't Room in Our Lives Now for Another Baby." Francke and her husband already had three children when she became pregnant again. She had just taken a full-time job; her husband was planning a career change; and their youngest had just started school. So there was just no room for a new baby in their lives. Francke experienced conflicting emotions, especially as she waited for the procedure to be performed. Her husband assured her that it was "not a life," but her body and mind knew otherwise. Following the abortion, she and her husband reminded each other that it made sense not to have a baby. Somewhat surprisingly, Francke described having a "very little ghost" thereafter that would appear whenever she saw something beautiful. The baby would wave at her, and Francke would wave at the baby, saying, "Of course, we have room."[1]

None of my post-abortive friends or acquaintances has described a ghost present with them, but almost all have expressed a loss, a sadness, or a life-changing experience that informs all of their subsequent work. The one exception among post-abortive women I have known maintained that her numerous abortions were entirely the right thing to do. She described no regret. She enjoyed significant professional success, while her struggles with alcoholism, depression, and anger were known to those close to her.

How can there be such differing reactions by women to their own abortions? On one level, it may be due to the understanding of self and the rights one possesses. Abortion is often promoted as a "woman's right," or a function of her autonomy, or self-governance.[2] *Autonomy* is derived from the Greek and means "self-rule." Tom Beauchamp and James Childress describe autonomy as one of the four principles of medical ethics.[3] It is the purview of individuals to choose for themselves what interventions can be done on their own bodies by medical professionals. Autonomy therefore needs to be coupled with true informed consent, so an individual can make good choices. That said, it is respect for the patient's autonomy that prevents another from intervening (in the case of adults deemed "decisional") even if the decision made is not one the medical professional thinks is appropriate or good.

Is this an accurate picture of abortion? Should abortion really be described as an act of "self-rule"? To have an abortion can be a decision made by one person—the pregnant woman. The abortion decision is made about another human being—the developing child. Further, abortion is a procedure that is carried out by another (or others)—the abortionist(s). Therefore, abortion is beyond an act of self-rule. It is an "over-other-rule" because it is an act of using a third party to overrule and destroy a defenseless other.

The Illusion of the Autonomous Mother

Abortion-as-an-act-of-autonomy is a misnomer for several reasons.[4] Autonomy—self-rule—does not give one person license to destroy another without cause. Second, autonomy does not necessitate a third party to do another's bidding. Third, autonomy should not degrade the medical profession into mere consumerism, for physicians have autonomy too. Yet that is not the way autonomy is practiced in the world we inhabit. In the claim that abortion is an act of autonomy, there can be really only one autonomous person: the pregnant woman.

A pregnant woman is a person in her own right, but she also temporarily houses another human body: the zygote, the embryo, and then the fetus—all names for the same baby, at sequential stages of development. Any obstetrician knows that he or she has at least two patients when a pregnant woman presents for consultation. Both the mother and the developing baby must be considered in matters of treatment, medications, and advice. Any medication the pregnant woman ingests or receives is shared with the baby as well. Some drugs can cause "serious, permanent or fatal side effects," including birth defects, and patients need to be warned of that possibility. The most stringent warning is the FDA's "black box warning," where a warning, outlined by a black border, is placed on a medication or medical device.[5] One such medication is Accutane, a drug used to treat certain severe acne. It can only be prescribed to women of child-bearing age under certain strict conditions, including a negative pregnancy test.[6]

Physicians and pharmacists are not the only ones aware that more than one patient is involved in any pregnancy; so are medical malpractice insurers. Malpractice insurance premiums charged to obstetricians reflect that reality. Medical malpractice claims usually have to be filed within two years of the "time of discovery," but that time does not start "until the injured party reaches the age of eighteen."[7] Obstetricians must pay for "tail coverage," a term that refers to the time during which they may be sued after they have provided care for the patient—in this case, the patient that was *in utero* twenty or so years before. It is clear that when a pregnant woman presents for care, there is always more than one patient present.

When a pregnant woman has an abortion, the procedure is done to remove the other, tiny human body from the special protection of the mother's uterus, or womb. She may see it as her right to do so, and some governments allow and even provide for that "right." Yet the abortion, like all medical procedures on a pregnant woman, has effects on two lives. One life, the nascent human being in the mother's womb, is destroyed. The tiny human being is then disposed of as medical waste, although some organs and tissues may be transferred to the market to be used for research. The other life—the mother's life—is usually not ended at that time, yet her life is changed by the pregnancy and the abortion—in some ways, permanently so.

Pregnancy changes a woman's body, and not only in shape or function. In addition to the obvious physical changes of pregnancy, there are changes at the molecular level. Cell-free fetal DNA circulates in the blood of pregnant women. It is the basis of the noninvasive prenatal screening for both chromosomal abnormalities and single gene disorders often performed at 12 to 13 weeks' gestation.[8] During pregnancy, there is also exchange of cells from the mother to the developing child, and vice versa. This is called *microchimerism*. The term for fetal cells in the mother is *fetal microchimerism*. Measurable fetal cells in maternal circulation have been found as early as seven weeks of gestation, and as late as twenty-seven years postpartum.[9] Some refer to this as the "biological legacy of pregnancy."[10]

How does fetal microchimerism pertain to abortion? It turns out that fetal cells are also transferred to the mother during "elective termination" or abortion—even more so than during a miscarriage.[11] One could consider this the "biological legacy of abortion." There is no procedure that reverses time so that it becomes as if the pregnancy had never happened. There is always some effect, even if not a "very little ghost."

In abortion as autonomy, only the pregnant woman is autonomous (barring coercion by family members or others). The pregnant woman is the one who makes the choice to have the abortion done—although, granted, this decision is probably not done lightly. She decides that the growing child within her must stop living. The developing child has no say in the matter, no defense, and no legal recourse. In no other setting is this the case. There is no other situation in the United States in which one person can decide that another must die, and the decision-maker have no legal repercussions for that decision. If a man or woman kills another person, the perpetrator is answerable in court for such action. If one hires a gunman (or woman) to kill someone, both the one who hired and the one hired are responsible for that action. In the case of armed police or military action, the actors are empowered by the State to use deadly force. That is also true in the arena of capital punishment. If a parent harms or kills a child who has been born, the parent is answerable for that crime. Only in the case of abortion can an adult (or emancipated minor) kill another human being. And it is not only legal, it is a business transaction. Again, it is the mother's decision. She, not the child, is the autonomous actor in abortion.

Interestingly, the autonomy claim of the mother regarding the child's body is temporary. The autonomy trump card of the mother depends on the geographical location of the child (pertinent legal considerations are beyond the scope of this chapter). As long as the child is an embryo or a fetus *in the womb,* the mother can legally claim autonomy over the body-within-her-body and have the child's life ended in abortion. Once the child is born, however, the woman's claim of autonomy extends only over her own body proper, not over the child's. How, then, is the exercise of the will of the woman over the person of the child an act of autonomy, "self-rule"? The claim of autonomy in this case errs in at least two ways. It is illusory: a cultural and legal fiction contrived to provide a solution to the problem of an unwelcome pregnancy. It is also a misapplication of the important concept of autonomy, for in fact it is "*other*-rule."

Neither is the abortionist autonomous. He or she functions primarily as a technician in this scenario. The abortion facilities exist to rid women of unwanted children before birth. The abortionist does not exist to provide care to either the pregnant woman or to her developing child. The abortionist's role is to destroy the developing child. If that does not happen, the abortion is unsuccessful. The abortionist is present to do the woman's bidding. Can the abortionist determine the hours of his or her availability? Presumably, yes. Yet the entire reason for his or her presence in the facility is to comply with the woman's stated desire. While the abortionist may facilitate the transfer of fetal parts to companies that use them for research, the main role of the abortionist is to perform abortions. If there were no market for providing abortions, abortionists would not have a purpose. In abortion, only the pregnant woman exercises *autonomy*. This does not, however, negate the abortionist's actions or moral culpability.

Further, abortion converts the profession of medicine into a consumerist business, although it is not the only procedure with this effect. The traditional Hippocratic Oath, which has been used by medical professionals for millennia, disallowed abortion. That is to say, those who professed to be Hippocratic physicians swore they would not perform abortions. More recent versions of the Hippocratic Oath often do not include such a prohibition. Instead, an elective abortion is often seen as a service provided to the one who seeks it. It is a service that can be purchased. Because the "providers" of abortion are licensed by the State, it is argued, abortion should be universally available. The Committee on Ethics of the American College of Obstetricians and Gynecologists (ACOG) reaffirmed in 2016 their 2007 "The Limits of Conscientious Refusal in Reproductive Medicine" (Number 385). Included in that document is this recommendation: "Physicians and other health care providers have the duty to refer patients in a timely manner to other providers if they do not feel that they can in conscience provide the standard reproductive services that patients request."[12] Note that it is the provision of *services requested* that ACOG requires to be done. This is a description of a consumer-provider relationship, with the pregnant woman as customer. The obstetrician is not an autonomous actor, according to the ACOG, but must provide the requested service, or else refer the woman to another "provider" who will do so. For the physician who cannot morally acquiesce to abortion, this is not autonomy at all. It is either submitting to tyranny or acting in complicity.

Nurses and abortion facility staff are also involved in abortions. Their experience has been described as "private and anguished ambivalence,"[13] as well as "nightmares of choice."[14] Additionally, a survey of seventy-five registered nurses working in labor and delivery areas of six California hospitals revealed criticism by coworkers for "both accepting and refusing patient care assignments" in cases of pregnancy termination.[15]

"Patients marked by liberty alone, without moral responsibility, can expect only technical services from professionals, no more," avers William F. May in *The Physician's Covenant*.[16] But are professionals, particularly physicians, merely technicians? Are "provider" and "physician" synonymous? Should they be? May finds the model of physician as technician lacking: "The bare negatives—'Do no harm,' 'Do no wrong,' and 'Respect autonomy'—fall short of the professional's positive obligations to serve the patient's well-being."[17] He argues for the understanding of a physician's responsibility toward his or her patient as covenantal, not contractual. May labels contracts as "external," with a limited time frame and the goal of expedience, in contrast to covenants. Covenants have more to do with the identity of the persons involved. A covenant is "grounded in the transcendent": a gift in recognition of a gift given. A covenant, according to May, results in both professional self-regulation and discipline, and fidelity to the patient.[18]

Edmund Pellegrino and David Thomasma, writing in *The Virtues in Medical Practice*, describe the relationship further. The physician is to be "the patient's advocate, and not simply an instrument of social, institutional, or fiscal policies."[19] Additionally they write, "In an ethic of trust, the physician is impelled to develop a relationship with the patient from the very outset that includes becoming familiar with who and what the patient is and how she wants to meet the serious challenges" of her life.[20] That is hardly the description of a "provider." Moreover, a physician treating a pregnant woman has two (or more, in the case of twins or greater multiples) patients to consider. The covenant extends to the preborn as well as to the adult.

That is not true of autonomy. Autonomy, in part a reaction to the flagrant paternalism of the past, is important. Coupled with truly informed consent, it gives the patient a voice, and provides protection from unwanted treatment. It is not, and cannot be, the trump card of life, however. As pointed out in the preceding discussion, autonomy for one person means, in the case of abortion, servitude, acquiescence, or destruction for others. There must be a better way. And, indeed, there is.

The Law of Creation

There is a law that predates Hippocrates, *autos-nomos,* and the Greeks themselves. It is the law of creation, of like begetting like, and the law of entities. It is an ancient law that began in a garden, and it continues to this day. It is a law that has not changed over the millennia of history. It is said that not one "jot" or "tittle" (Matt. 5:18 NKJV) of it will change while the earth remains. A *jot* is equivalent to the smallest letter in the Greek alphabet, the *iota,*[21] whereas the *tittle* is equivalent to the dot over the letter, *i,* or the size of the period at the end of a sentence.[22]

The Genesis account reveals the Creator of the universe creating humankind—male and female—in the image of God (Gen. 1:26–27). That image, the *imago Dei*, persists in all succeeding generations of human beings all around the globe. What does it mean to be made in God's image? Many excellent thinkers down through the ages have applied themselves to this question. Augustine identified the image of the triune God in humankind in terms of intellect, memory, and will.[23] Thomas Aquinas saw the image of God reflected in the mind of "intellectual creatures."[24] Anthony Hoekema interprets the image through the root meanings of Hebrew words used: *tselem* ("to carve") and *demuth* ("to be like").[25] Millard Erickson in *Christian Theology* explains that the image of God is about who we are, not some feature we possess or something we do. He writes, "Whatever sets humans apart from the rest of creation, they alone are capable of having a conscious personal relationship with the Creator and of responding to him, can know God and understand what he desires of them, can love, worship, and obey their Maker. These responses most completely fulfill the Maker's intention for the human. The human also has an eternal dimension."[26]

The Genesis creation account includes God forming creatures that would reproduce "according to their kind." After creating humans—both male and female—in His own image, God blesses them and commands them to "be fruitful and multiply" (Gen. 1:21–28). Birds produce birds; cattle produce cattle; humans produce humans: each after their kind. It is a matter of our nature. A pregnant woman is not just reproducing a "clump of cells." Whether it is a zygote or an embryo the size of a full-stop at the end of a sentence, or a full-term fetus about to be born, the being is undeniably human, and it is a human being distinct from the mother.

Linda Bird Francke discovered this while she was situated in a small waiting area before her abortion. She described herself as "alone with my microscopic baby." Even though her husband had insisted that "it" was not a life but rather "a bunch of cells smaller than [his] fingernail," she knew the truth. She described it this way: "Any woman who has had children knows that certain feeling in her taut, swollen breasts, and the slight but constant ache in her uterus that signals the arrival of a life."[27]

Yet, the abortion proceeded.

Abortion is but a modern version of the Solomonic sword actually wielded. Two women came to that wisest of kings, each claiming one baby as her own (1 Kings 3:16–28). King Solomon asked for a sword, in order to cut the baby in half and give each woman a share. One of the women agreed with that plan; the other implored the king not to divide the baby, but to give the living child to the other woman. The king saw clearly that the woman who sought not to hurt the child was the real mother, and her baby was restored to her.

In pregnancy, two lives claim (for a brief period of time) one body. The one with a voice agrees with the abortionist that the sword (or suction curettage, or medication) must be wielded in order to solve the problem. Money is paid, and the deed is done.

What should we have learned from the judgment of Solomon? F. W. Boreham explicates some vital lessons one can learn from this ancient story.[28] One is the difference between *quantities* and *entities.* A quantity is something that can be divided without doing it harm. Boreham gives the examples of a ton of coal, a quart of milk, and a pound of butter. All of these quantities can be divided into two parts without harm to the coal, the milk, or the butter. Entities, however, are different: a song, a beautiful painting, or a rose could not be divided into two parts without being damaged or destroyed. Boreham writes, "These things—and all the best things in life—are *Entities*;

they are like the baby at the city gate; you can only divide them by destroying them."[29]

In the realm of *Entities*, Boreham advises, mathematics becomes unreliable:

> Solomon proves it at the city gate. It may be true that half a sovereign and half a sovereign make a sovereign; it is obviously untrue that a half a baby and half a baby make a baby. Let the sword do its deadly work; let it cleave this baby into two parts; and half a baby plus half a baby will represent but the grim and gruesome mockery of a baby. Two halves of a baby make no baby at all.
>
> On this higher plane of human sentiment and experience, the laws of Mathematics collapse completely.[30]

Mathematics is not reliable in abortion, either. Two minus the destruction of one does not result in one whole autonomous remainder. We know this is true from Scripture. Returning to the Genesis account, the second generation of humanity reveals in part the law of harvesting (Gen. 4:1–15). Cain, out of jealousy, kills Abel. That is not the end of the story. Abel's blood cries out to God from the ground, and God hears that injustice. Cain is subsequently cursed from the ground, which will no longer "yield its strength" to him (Gen. 4:12 NKJV). Proverbs 22:8 confirms that the one who sows wrongdoing will reap calamity. This truth is reiterated in the New Testament, where we are warned against being deceived: whatever we sow, we shall also reap—because God is not mocked (Gal. 6:7).

We know this is true from collected data. An important study from New Zealand was published in the *British Journal of Psychiatry* in 2008. It was a thirty-year longitudinal study of a birth cohort of children in New Zealand with this finding: "Women who had had abortions had rates of mental health problems that were about 30% higher than rates of disorder in other women. Although rates of all forms of disorder were higher in women exposed to abortion, the conditions most associated with abortion included anxiety disorders and substance use disorders." Remarkably, the authors concluded that "the overall effects of abortion on mental health proved to be small." While a 30 percent increased risk for mental health disorders is certainly not evidence to be dismissed lightly, an even more telling conclusion followed. The study's authors conceded that "there is nothing in this study that would suggest that the termination of pregnancy was associated with lower risks of mental health problems than birth following an unwanted pregnancy."[31] For those arguing for abortion based on the mental health needs of the mother, this longitudinal study offers zero support.

We also know about the mental health risks from experience. Each of my post-abortive friends has been changed by the experience of abortion. They are not alone. Responses to abortion tend to fall into three primary categories, whatever the circumstances surrounding the event may have been. It certainly may have seemed the only or the best option at the time, but the rearview mirror often offers a different view. One possibility is to recognize that the act of abortion has destroyed another human being's life, and thus to seek forgiveness and redemption from God, the Author of all of our lives, and the Forgiver of all of our sin. Another possibility is to recognize the effect of abortion on the unborn, but to neglect or refuse to ask forgiveness, and to live with the guilt that ensues. A third is to deny that abortion is a wrong, or even a problem, and to tell yourself that repeatedly for the rest of your life.

The Law of Christ

However important the principle of autonomy may be in the practice of medicine, it is not a biblical concept. The New Testament affirms the law of creation and explicates the law of Christ. It was Jesus Christ, one of the trinitarian Godhead, who took on the flesh of humankind. In that cloak of flesh, He healed many, washed the feet of His disciples—including the one who would soon betray Him—and died a cruel and totally undeserved death to pay the penalty for the sin of every human being. This same Jesus said, "Whoever wants to be my disciple must deny themselves and take up their cross and follow me" (Mark 8:34 NIV).[32] He taught His disciples, "Anyone who wants to be first must be the very last, and the servant of all" (Mark 9:35). That is hardly a description of autonomy!

Regarding rights, Paul teaches that not everything which is a right is beneficial (1 Cor. 6:12). He instructs believers that our "bodies are members of Christ himself" (1 Cor. 6:15). Further, he writes that we are to honor God with our bodies, because we have been bought with a price (1 Cor. 6:20). Our bodies "are temples of the Holy Spirit" (1 Cor. 6:19). Paul points out that he did not avail himself of all of his rights in his dealings with the Corinthians (1 Cor. 9:1–23). Moreover, Paul argues that while one may have a "right to do anything," not everything is beneficial or constructive (1 Cor. 10:23). Indeed, we are instructed to seek the good of others (1 Cor. 10:24). This is not Paul's example only: he is following the "example of Christ" (1 Cor. 11:1). Similarly, Paul tells his readers that "none of us lives for ourselves alone" (Rom. 14:7). He instructs the Philippian believers, "Do nothing out of selfish ambition or vain conceit" (Phil. 2:3). Rather, they (and we) should look not to our own interests, but to the interests of others (Phil. 2:4). To the Galatian Christians, Paul calls this the "law of Christ" (Gal. 6:2), and it is a far cry from autonomy.

Conclusion

It should come as no surprise, then, that abortion as an act of autonomy has no winners. In its wake are only victims. The unborn are converted into parts for research (not to mention dollars) or medical waste. The blood of millions of these innocents cries out to the Creator God, whose ear is attuned to injustice. Yet they are not the only victims of abortion. Whether abortions occur by autonomy or through coercion, mothers, too, are victims. They carry with them throughout their lives far more than fetal cells. Physicians are transformed into perpetrators or complicit technicians, and the physician-patient relationship becomes nothing more than a consumer-driven contract. Nurses and staff of abortion centers are caught up in the lucrative enterprise, and they bear their own scars. It is ironic that the choice of *autonomy*—self-rule—leaves so many victims in its wake.

8

Marvelously Revealed: The Symphony of a Woman's Body

—Donna Harrison—

One of the most joyful exhibits at our local county fair is the "Wonders of Birth" barn. Local farmers plan ahead to have cows, goats, chickens, and other farm animals give birth at the time of the fair. It is always the most popular exhibit of the entire fairgrounds. Even the most hardened of old-timers smile at the kids who are in awe of the process of birth. "How did that little cow get in there?" is the question asked every year.

As an OB-GYN, I have spent most of my professional life thinking about procreation. And as a woman, wife, and mother of nine, with five living children, I have experienced personally many of the joys and griefs that accompany the gift of procreation. In this chapter I want to share with you some of the wonder and awe that comes with considering some of the nuances of this tremendous gift of procreation, which connects us in flesh to both the past and the future of humanity.

The Community of Human Beings and the Uniqueness of Being Female

What makes up the community of human beings? While that seems like a very simple question, the answer has profound implications. We are part of the community of human beings because we are human. What makes us human? Being born of human parents, starting at the time of fertilization, and continuing on in one continuous existence until our death. This is biological reality. We all breathe, eat, and move. We have unique capacities to think, run, walk, cry, love, react, and communicate. These are aspects of the gifts God has given to all human beings. One of the gifts is what is written into our chromosomes. Humans have chromosomes that are common to all human beings, whether male or female. These chromosomes make us human and determine how our human body functions.

Being human gives us a common identity with all other human beings. Yet in the area of procreation, we are male or female. We don't become a female by dressing in female clothes, or by altering our bodies to fit some constantly varying abstract idea of what society at the time considers to be feminine. Our body itself is either female or male at the time of our first beginning as a human being. The reality of being male or female is written into every cell of our body at the time of our creation as a human being, that is, at the time of fertilization.

Whether we are male or female depends on whether an X chromosome in the sperm cell from our father fertilizes our mother's egg, or a Y chromosome from our father fertilizes our mother's egg.

If the sperm from our father contains a Y chromosome as one of the chromosomes we receive from our father, we are male. If the sperm from our father contains an X chromosome as one of the chromosomes we receive from our father, we are female. It is as simple as that biological fact. And this biological fact determines our role in bringing into life the next generation of human beings. It is our X or Y chromosome that defines our role in procreation. And this is where the fabulous symphony of a woman's body is marvelously revealed.

The Symphony of a Woman's Body in Procreation

God not only provides for the creation of the next generation of human beings at the point of sperm egg membrane fusion (fertilization) but also writes into that moment the compassion of His care and forethought by designing that event to take place in a special place of protection and nurture. And that unique place of protection and nurture for the beginning of human beings is within the womb of a woman. So let us take a closer look at the way God wrote His image in creation by looking at how He designed the woman's body to function in the procreation, protection, and provision for the next generation of humanity.

How a Woman's Body Prepares for Procreation

The symphony of human creation is an amazing coordination of the bodies of both the husband and the wife in order to bring new human life into the world in the most protected and nurturing way possible. Self-giving, protection, and love outline the context of the creation of new human life. This self-giving, protection, and love are sung into existence in a woman's body.

When a girl is still in her mother's womb, her tiny body has within it the egg cells that she will have in adulthood, in fact millions more than she will ever use in her life. And her womb is also formed while she is still in her mother's womb. When a female baby is born, her ovaries still contain millions of egg cells. Throughout her childhood, most of these egg cells disappear, so that by the time she reaches puberty, only the best are left. Still, she has thousands of these immature egg cells waiting for a special signal from her brain to start preparing for possible fertilization.

When a girl reaches the start of puberty—usually between the ages of twelve and sixteen—a special place in her brain, the hypothalamus, starts to send wake-up signals to her ovaries. These chemical messages tell the ovaries to start the process of maturing batches of eggs, of which (usually) one egg per month will be released and possibly fertilized.

As her ovaries respond to the message from her brain, her ovaries start to make special hormones that cause the lining of her womb to grow. If there is no new human being formed that month, then the signals from her brain slow down, the lining of her womb sloughs off, and she has a *period,* which is the lining of the womb leaving her body. Let's look in a little more detail at this process, to grasp the fabulous wonder of this hormone symphony.

First of all, we have to know how to count the measures of this symphony. We can keep track of what is going on in our body by looking at what our body is doing, over and over again. To make things easier to count, we call *cycle day 1* the day that we first see bleeding from our period. Our cycle starts on that day and ends on the first day we see bleeding from the next period. For most women, the next period will start somewhere between 26 to 32 days later.

Let's consider the awesome things that are happening while a woman's body plays out the song started by her brain.

Remember that the woman's brain conducts this symphony. Her brain starts the messages drummed out by the hypothalamus. We do not know exactly how the hypothalamus knows to start these messages, but we do know that the hypothalamus has the ability to sense what is going on in the woman's body, and at what point she is in her cycle by sensing the hormone levels in her blood.

Depending on what her hypothalamus senses, it will send signals to her pituitary gland, the master gland located in the base of her brain. The pituitary gland then sends messages to her ovary. These special messages from the pituitary are either FSH (follicle stimulating hormone), which is the message given from her pituitary to her ovary in the first half of her cycle; or LH (luteinizing hormone), which is the message her pituitary sends to her ovary in the second half of her cycle. And these messages tell her ovary what to do!

A woman's ovaries are the place where new eggs are getting ready for possible fertilization. When her ovaries get the FSH signal, they start allowing her eggs to get ready. The eggs get ready inside a fluid sac called a "follicle." So now you can understand why the hormone that tells the eggs to get ready is called the follicle stimulating hormone. The ovary takes the FSH orders from the pituitary and gets the eggs ready for release and possible fertilization.

Just as important as the eggs getting ready is what the follicle sac itself is doing. As the eggs grow, the follicle cells make another important hormone called "estradiol." Estradiol causes the lining cells of the womb to start growing fast, to make a lush place for the new human being to grow. This all happens from day 1 (the first day of her last period) to approximately day 14, when the egg is released. That is why the first half of the woman's cycle is called the "follicular phase."

Then, when the woman's brain (hypothalamus) senses in her blood that enough estradiol has been made, the hypothalamus sends out the other, different signal called the luteinizing hormone. When the ovary receives the LH orders, two amazing things happen. The first is that the ovary releases the egg, which is now ready to be fertilized. The egg is swept into the waiting fallopian tube, which connects the ovary to the womb. If the egg will be fertilized, it will be fertilized in the fallopian tube, and this must take place within twenty-four hours. If it is not fertilized in that timeframe, the egg will disintegrate.

The second amazing response is that the follicle that released the egg now becomes a factory to produce a very important hormone called "progesterone." Progesterone is key to everything that happens from here. You can remember the name "progesterone" by knowing what the parts of this name mean. *Pro* means "for." *Gest* refers to "gestation," which means pregnancy. And *sterone* refers to the fact that it is a steroid hormone. So, *pro-gest-sterone* means "for-pregnancy-hormone." It is progesterone that changes a woman's body to be able to receive and nurture her son or daughter within her womb. Progesterone causes the lush lining to make the hundreds of cellular changes that have to happen to allow the embryo to implant.[1] And how much progesterone a woman's ovary makes is directly related to how much LH signal comes from her pituitary. It is an amazing symphony!

Even more amazing, the pituitary keeps sending LH throughout the second half of a woman's cycle. But if she does not have an embryo formed during that second half of the cycle, the LH signal from the pituitary stops, causing progesterone to stop being produced in the ovary factory. When progesterone stops being produced, then the lining of the woman's womb starts to break down.

She may feel tense and moody due to the fall in progesterone. Eventually, the lining of her womb sheds and she has her period. Then the whole cycle starts again.

That is a simple description of a fabulously complex symphony happening every month in a woman's cycle. But something else even more amazing happens in the woman's body when a new human being is created: the woman's body realizes this and changes almost immediately to accommodate the presence of her embryonic son or daughter!

The Song of Fertilization

It may be surprising, but sperm cells from a man's body cannot immediately fertilize a woman's egg. These sperm cells have to change to be able to fertilize, and that change actually happens a few hours after being exposed to a woman's body. Sperm cells continue to live in the woman's body and are capable of fertilizing her egg for up to five days. Look at how amazing that is! Sperm cells are the only human cells that are made in one person's body but are designed to live and do their work in another person's body!

In about the middle of a woman's cycle, the part of a woman's womb called the fallopian tube starts to sweep over the ovary and prepares to receive the egg once it is released. Once the egg is released, it is swept into the fallopian tube, and that is where the egg might be fertilized. Remember that a woman's egg cell is able to be fertilized only within twenty-four hours after being released from her ovary. If her egg cell is not fertilized in that time, it will not be able to make a new human being. So, the woman's body has been designed to nurture the sperm cells for several days while they are waiting for her egg to be released. When her egg is released, often the egg encounters millions of sperm cells that try to penetrate through the cumulus oophorus, the protective layer around the egg.

The first sperm cell to penetrate the egg causes a chemical spark (or the closing of zinc channels) that keeps any other sperm cell from being able to penetrate the egg.

Once the cell membranes of that sperm cell and that egg cell have come together, the sperm no longer exists, and the egg no longer exists. What does exist is a new human being, a one-celled embryo called a zygote.[2] This zygote grows and divides into a two-celled embryo, then a four-celled embryo, and so on. And, while it is growing and dividing, the embryo is being rolled down the mother's fallopian tube toward her womb by tiny hairs on the ends of the cells that line the fallopian tube. This rolling action prepares the embryo to get ready to implant once he or she arrives in the mother's womb. Interestingly, this rolling action is also controlled by the hormone progesterone, which is made by the mother's ovary. And remember, progesterone is also at the same time getting her womb ready to receive and nourish the embryo.

Once the embryo reaches her mother's womb, the embryo begins to snuggle into the rich lining of her mother's womb, which immediately provides a covering of protection and nourishment. The cells of the embryo that form the placenta begin to weave their way between her mother's blood vessels in the lining of the womb, giving the baby nourishment and taking away the waste products from the baby's body.

So what happens when the pituitary starts shutting down the LH signal at the end of the cycle? Does the progesterone production factory in the ovary shut down? No, God has already taken care of this problem. Within days of the embryo forming, the embryo begins a chemical "cross-talk" with the mother's body using a chemical called human chorionic gonadotropin (hCG). The embryo produces increasing amounts of hCG, especially after he or she implants in his or her mother's womb. This hCG tells the mother's body that her preborn child is here, growing in her womb. The hCG signal tells the mother's ovaries to keep making progesterone, to keep the baby alive. It is the continuous production of progesterone by the mother's ovary that continues to change the mother's body to enable her to nourish and protect her embryo as he or she grows.

These are only the beginning of wonderful changes that happen in a woman's body when she becomes pregnant. The hormones of pregnancy not only affect a woman's womb, but also affect her brain, her breasts, her ovaries, and her immune system.

Changes in a Woman's Brain

As you know, the woman's brain is always sensing and aware of the hormones that her body is making. As the baby implants in the mother's womb, he or she starts to make the chemical hCG. This is the same chemical that leads to a positive pregnancy test in the mother's urine. The woman's brain senses the presence of hCG and stops making FSH and LH, the signals that we talked about in the first part of this chapter. So, the woman does not release any more eggs, and also doesn't have any periods.

Some fascinating research has brought to light the presence of a baby's cells in the mother's bloodstream. This research implies that some of these cells stay around in certain parts of the mother's body, a phenomenon called *microchimerism*.[3] While this field of research is still developing, the idea brings potential new meaning to the concept of a "one flesh" relationship!

Changes in a Woman's Immune System

You might know that when a person has a transplant of a kidney or heart or some other organ, the person who received the transplant sometimes has to take drugs to prevent his or her body from "rejecting" the transplanted organ. That is because our bodies recognize things that are "not our body," and then our body mounts an immune response against that foreign tissue. So the obvious question is: *Why doesn't our body reject our preborn children?*

The answer again, as in most things about pregnancy, is progesterone. This hormone causes a woman's body to not mount an immune response against her preborn child. Progesterone seems to be acting directly at the level of the immune cells in the woman's womb to cause this kind of "tolerance." This is another fabulous example of how women are designed to respond to their preborn children with an environment that loves and nurtures and does not reject their presence.

Changes in a Woman's Breast[4]

A girl before puberty has very little breast tissue. In puberty, under the stimulation of the hormone estrogen made by her ovaries, a girl's breasts begin to grow. But the type of breast tissue that she grows is called type 1 and type 2 tissue. It is an immature tissue that cannot make milk. It is the kind of tissue from which 99 percent of breast cancer arises.

When a woman carries a baby for the first time, the organ that feeds the baby—the placenta—starts to make special hormones that change the mother's breast. In the first half of pregnancy, the placenta makes estrogen. This hormone causes a woman's breast tissue to grow rapidly, which is why she experiences tenderness. But this rapidly growing tissue is immature "stem cell" tissue called type 1 and type 2 tissue. This type of breast tissue grows rapidly, but it cannot make milk.

After a mom carries her baby into the second half of pregnancy, the placenta makes a new set of growth hormones that change the immature type 1 and type 2 breast tissue into type 4 tissue, which is tissue that can make milk. Type 4 tissue is *permanently cancer resistant.*

No breast cancers arise from type 4 tissue. These hormones begin to be produced after the woman is halfway through her pregnancy (around 20 weeks of gestation). By the time the baby reaches 32 weeks of gestation, about half of the mother's breast tissue has been changed from cancer-prone type 1 and type 2 tissue into cancer-resistant type 4 tissue. By the time a woman reaches the end of her pregnancy, about 95 percent of her breast is now type 4 tissue. This is a fabulous design that causes a mother to be able to feed her baby when the baby is born! After she stops breastfeeding, the type 4 tissue becomes type 3 tissue. But the good news is that type 3 tissue is also permanently cancer resistant.

Equally wondrous, when a woman breastfeeds her baby, her body releases a powerful bonding hormone called *oxytocin,* which causes the milk to flow. And it is oxytocin that is known to be involved in emotional bonding.

Once we understand, as women, that our bodies are a gift where the next generation originates, we can begin to understand some of the ways in which mistreating that gift has consequences that reach far into the future.

Physical Consequences of Intentionally Ending the Lives of Our Preborn Children

As an OB-GYN, I have never encountered a patient who became pregnant for the purpose of getting an abortion. And I have never heard of any doctor in this field who had such a patient. Abortion is not something that any woman desires. It is a last resort, a kind of desperate attempt to use surgery to solve a social or situational problem. Those problems are real. The circumstances that lead a woman to contemplate abortion are real. But the question is whether or not killing our children within our womb is the best solution to solving them. As a physician and a researcher, and as a woman and mother, I would argue that killing our children is not the best answer. Abortion leaves one victim (our child) dead and the other (ourselves) wounded. Yet, the abortion industry markets to our fear and tells us that we can turn back the clock if we just take a few pills, or submit to the D&C. What they don't talk about are long-term consequences for us. And that is what I want to talk about in this next section.

Killing Our Preborn Children Increases Our Risk of Breast Cancer[5]

Not all breast cancer is from abortion. And not all abortions increase a woman's risk of breast cancer. But when we understand the way our breast was designed to grow, mature, and function, it is simple to understand why ending the lives of our preborn children increases breast cancer risk, especially if we had those abortions before we ever brought a child to term. This is easy to understand when you realize how a pregnancy affects a woman's breast, changing her breast from cancer-susceptible tissue in the first half of her pregnancy to milk-producing, cancer-resistant tissue in the second half of her pregnancy. But what happens when you interrupt her pregnancy before that tissue transformation has had a chance to take place?

If a woman has never carried a pregnancy past 32 weeks, her breast is filled with mostly cancer-susceptible type 1 and 2 tissue. When that woman becomes pregnant and then loses a child for any reason—whether by accident, infection/illness, or elective abortion (the most common reason in this country)—her breast is arrested in a state where most of the breast tissue is cancer susceptible. Her ultimate risk will depend on two factors: how much cancer-susceptible type 1 and 2 tissue she has in her breast, and how long she carries that cancer-susceptible tissue before she matures it into type 4 cancer-resistant tissue.

So, for example, if a woman has had one pregnancy she carries to term, and then she aborts her next pregnancy, she is unlikely to see much of an increase in her lifetime risk of breast cancer. This is because when she carried her first pregnancy to term, 95 percent of her breast tissue was permanently changed into type 3 and 4 tissue. Type 3 and 4 tissue is *permanently* cancer resistant. It is only the remaining 5 percent of her breast tissue that is still cancer susceptible. So, even though another pregnancy caused a little bit of increase in that remaining 5 percent of type 1 and 2 tissue, overall most of her breast tissue remains cancer-resistant type 3 and 4 tissue. However, if a woman has two abortions before she ever brings a baby to term, and if she delays having that full-term baby until she is in her thirties, she has increased her lifetime risk of breast cancer because she has increased the total amount of cancer-susceptible type 1 and 2 tissue, and she has carried that susceptible tissue for a long time.

So, in brief, all the risk factors for breast cancer boil down basically to two major questions: (1) How much cancer-susceptible type 1 and 2 tissue do I have in my breast? The more cancer susceptible tissue, the higher a woman's lifetime risk. And, (2) how long have I carried cancer-susceptible type 1 and type 2 tissue in my breast before maturing that tissue into cancer-resistant, milk-producing type 3 and 4 tissue? The longer a woman delays carrying a baby to term, the higher her risk. That is why women who have never had children have an increased risk of breast cancer. Carrying an unborn child to term is the single most important factor in lowering a woman's risk of breast cancer!

Killing Our Preborn Children Increases Our Risk of Preterm Birth[6]

Preterm birth is one of the greatest causes of death in newborn children. And the rate of preterm birth in the United States has steadily risen since the 1970s. Many researchers over the past fifty years have studied this trend. In fact, there are more than 160 scientific studies clearly demonstrating that women who have elective abortions are at increased risk of having premature babies in future pregnancies, especially babies born at the edge of being able to survive outside of the womb (22–26 weeks' gestation). There are two likely reasons this is so:

1. Our wombs were designed to stay closed until the baby is mature enough to survive outside of our womb. When a woman has an abortion, the strong tissue surrounding the opening of the womb can be damaged when the womb is forced open to remove the parts of the baby. This damage to the strong connective tissue of the cervix can be permanent and result in the inability of the womb in future pregnancies to carry a baby to maturity.
2. When a baby is aborted, there can be fragments of the baby's placental tissue that remains inside the womb, setting up a chronic infection, which can lead to preterm birth.

Killing Our Preborn Children Increases Our Risk of Suicide, Drug Abuse, and Major Depression[7]

A well-designed prospective study from New Zealand looked at mental health outcomes of women who aborted unwanted, unplanned pregnancies and compared these to women who brought unwanted, unplanned pregnancies to birth. What they discovered is that women who aborted their unwanted babies had greater subsequent mental health challenges than women who brought their unwanted babies to birth. The women who aborted faced more suicide, more drug abuse, and more depression. And this trend has been confirmed in other studies.

Why would women who abort their unwanted children do worse than women who bring their unwanted children to birth? We are created to bond to our children. Even women who face situations where they can't imagine taking care of a baby still at some level bond to their baby. Breaking that bond hurts. We can deny the hurt, we can ignore the hurt, but the hurt is still there.

I have taken care of women who cry about their abortion even thirty years later. The death of any child, born or preborn, changes us. And every one of our children who die are human beings who have a relationship to us.

The abortion industry lies to women and says, "If you have this abortion, then it will be just like you were never pregnant." The truth is that once you are pregnant, you are a mother. You cannot become "never pregnant." You will become either the mother of a living child or the mother of a dead child. And those consequences are irrevocable. Both routes change your life forever. One route brings incredible joy. The other brings incredible sorrow, often to the mother, and always to the heart of the One who created that child. Both routes are permanent. And both choices change the history of our world forever.

When we intentionally kill our preborn children in abortion, we end the life not only of that son or daughter, but also their children and grandchildren who will never exist. Each of us are part of the fabric of human life, woven together as children, spouses, aunts, uncles, grandparents, nieces, nephews, and so on. Our children are not only in relationship to us, but to their father, their grandparents, their siblings, and extended family members. None of us lives as our own. And none of us dies as our own. While we live, we are responsible for the lives that God has given us to care for, no matter how inconvenient or challenging they are to us. As Christians, we embrace meaning in suffering and inconvenience, a meaning that takes us out of ourselves as the sole purpose of our lives and places us in a self-giving, loving relationship with the other human beings in our lives.

Regret and Forgiveness

When driving to work, I would frequently pass a simple black-and-white billboard: "All saints have a past. All sinners have a future." Many of us women have done things we look back on with deep regret. That is why there are so many ministries available to help women with post-abortion regret.[8] The regret is real. The mother is the second victim of her abortion. If you are a family member or friend of someone suffering from post-abortion regret, help her find a safe place where she can talk and go through the steps needed for her healing. You may save her life.

Conclusion

I hope this chapter has given you a glimpse of the fabulous design of a woman's body, and the gift that we have been given to participate in the future of the world, through making a place for life to develop. I hope you can cherish this gift and use it wisely, appreciating what a wonderful creation you are.

CLAIM 4

I Should Not Have to Raise an Unwanted Child

9

The Myth of the Unwanted Child: How Adoption Powerfully Dispels the Lie

—Bethany Bomberger—

Social media is chock-a-block full of gender reveals featuring confetti blasters, mysteries unveiled in pink or blue filled cakes, and happy women sharing about their pregnancies. But I know that often a woman is met with fear and trepidation when she discovers the news of her pregnancy. As a woman whose first pregnancy was not under ideal circumstances, I understand some of these sentiments.

Honestly, it is hard even to articulate all the emotions that surface when the news of something so life-changing occurs. After the shock wears off, there can be many reasons why a woman feels a sense of "I don't want this!" "I can't handle this!" "This wasn't part of my plan!" Pro-abortion advocates take advantage of this fear and uncertainty and, instead of helping moms understand the loving options of parenting and adoption, they offer abortion. This seeming quick fix is justified with reasoning that may sound somewhat innocuous at first—"Every child should be wanted." But ultimately this approach adds trauma to distress.

Adding brokenness to brokenness never brings healing. God never gets tired of redeeming, renewing, and creating beauty from ashes. He never gets tired of passionately pursuing His creation because He knows our worth—even when others can't see it. Abortion is never a better option than adoption. Abortion is rooted in fear and leads to physical, emotional, and spiritual destruction. Adoption is rooted in love and leads to a future and a hope. As Christians who have personal relationships with the Author of hope and love, we are called to be on the forefront of the adoption movement.

The Myth of the Unwanted Child

The myth of the unwanted child is ages old. But I want to take you back, for a moment, to a pivotal time when the motto "Every Child a Wanted Child" became an anthem woven into the fabric of our society. We all know the 1920s were affectionately called the Roaring Twenties. They were marked by the sounds of jazz bands and voices like the celebrated Louis Armstrong. Women's fashion brought flapper dresses with beads and sequins. Men wore suits with suspenders, bow ties, and Great Gatsby-like styles. Gelatin molds were all the rage. The end of WWI had ushered in a booming economy, and the fragrance of freedom (for some) was in the air. America was rapidly becoming a place where hardworking men and women could see their dreams come to fruition. The passing of the landmark Nineteenth Amendment to the Constitution officially allowed women the right to vote. America was changing.

Unfortunately, in the drive for independence and a new sense of self-actualization, a number of severely misguided women began to emerge as leaders. On a quest to define feminism, these leaders began to sway culture and attempt to solve problems in poverty-stricken communities by promoting birth control and determining which unborn human beings had the right to be born. Margaret Sanger, the mother of the birth control movement, was motivated by the belief that only some humans were worthy of life. Steeped in eugenic racism (as evidenced by a multitude of Sanger's writings), birth control's main aim was "nothing more or less than the facilitation of the process of weeding out the unfit, of preventing the birth of defectives or of those who will become defectives."[1] This declaration in her book *Women and the New Race* (1920) is one of hundreds of examples from Sanger expressing her conviction that birth control had nothing to do with women's rights or of providing actual solutions to poverty. It was about crushing unseen purpose.

Part of this burgeoning movement actually began in 1917 with the production and printing of Margaret Sanger's *Birth Control Review*. The cover of the magazine's November 1923 issue illuminates her disturbing belief system and the motivation for her life's work. The featured sketch shows a distraught woman whose ankle is shackled to a large iron ball inscribed with the words "Unwanted Babies." This distressing image brings to life one of the most accepted slogans of the abortion industry.

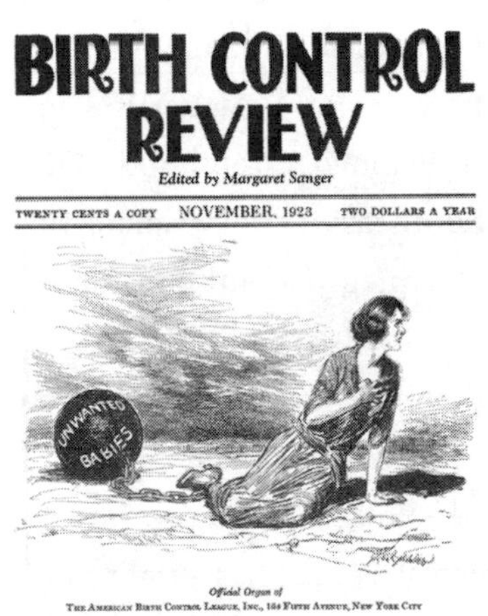

Throughout the 1900s the motto of Planned Parenthood (formerly known as the American Birth Control League), as printed on the back of their pamphlets, was "Every Child a Wanted Child." In Sanger's *Women and the New Race,* she writes: "Each and every unwanted child is likely to be in some way a social liability. It is only the wanted child who is likely to be a social asset."[2] Whoa. As a mama to four amazing kiddos (three of which could be considered "humanly unplanned") and as someone who has had the opportunity to teach hundreds of students over the years, I cannot help but find this line of thought incredibly disturbing. This slogan advocates the self-glorifying perspective that we, as mothers (and fathers), are able to determine a human being's value and ability to succeed based on the subjective quality of "wantedness."

The abortion industry champions this hopeless rhetoric, perpetuating the lie that only those humans who are wanted are worthy of life. Today, Sanger is praised by pro-abortion advocates for being the founder of modern day Planned Parenthood, the nation's leading abortion chain. The original slogan continues to be PP's unofficial motto. Pro-abortion advocates parrot this lie. It is at the core of Planned Parenthood's DNA, as seen in Planned Parenthood of Southeast Pennsylvania's mission statement until August 2020. "Planned Parenthood Southeastern Pennsylvania believes that every child should be a wanted child."[3] In a 2016 article, PP praises their "founder and reproductive rights trailblazer," saying: "Sanger was a true visionary. In her lifetime, she convinced Americans and people around the world that they have basic human rights: that every woman has a right to control her body, and *every child should be wanted and loved*; that all people should be able to decide when or whether to have a child and are entitled to sexual pleasure and fulfillment."[4] Sadly, this reasoning plays on the fear of the unknown in pregnancy and attempts to justify the principle that "every *unwanted* child should be a *dead* child."

Purpose from Day One

I offer this history lesson not just to take a glance back in time. It is important for understanding an industry that is predicated on deception and false marketing as it touts its position as the savior of the community and the champion of freedom. The Myth of the Unwanted Child perpetuates the lie that freedom comes when we choose to end another human being's life for our own benefit. This devalues humanity at every age and stage. It allows for a culture of death that accepts abortion, infanticide, euthanasia, and assisted suicide. When we think we can play God, we deny humanity's need for a Savior who comes to give life. He created us and remains ready to rescue and redeem our lives from our sinful choices. His heart is that we know our worth in Him and, in His strength, find hope in seeming hopelessness.

As Christians, we know that we were created with love and purpose. Psalm 139:13 so eloquently says, "You made all the delicate, inner parts of my body and knit me together in my mother's womb" (NLT). He took His time and care to fashion us in *His* image (Gen. 1:26). Our very existence gives us undeniable and irrevocable value. This is the revelation that I pray for every person, that they might see and understand that we carry the image of God within us. Sharing this eternal truth is the motivation for my life's work.

My husband Ryan and I run a nonprofit called the Radiance Foundation.[5] Our mission is to *illuminate* the intrinsic value of each individual person—"planned" or "unplanned." So, we *educate* audiences about a myriad of social issues in the context of God-given purpose. Our prayer is that we *motivate* people to put their knowledge and faith into action. One facet of our work has been to help raise funds (as speakers at fundraiser events) for pregnancy resource centers and maternity homes established to help women who are facing unplanned pregnancies. This has given us amazing opportunities to tour hundreds of pregnancy centers and maternity homes where we have been able to spend time with their directors, staff, and clients. We have seen, firsthand, their attractive counseling rooms, their ultrasound and nurse consultation facilities, their "Earn While You Learn" parenting classes, their baby and mama boutiques, and the vast number of other resources these centers and homes make available to families in need. The goal of these organizations is to help mothers and fathers see beyond their temporary fears so they can choose the life-affirming solutions of parenting or adoption. The staff and supporters are passionate about creating a culture of life by assisting families who may otherwise choose abortion. God works through these volunteers and staff members as they teach women and men to find value in every human life, including their own. They impart to them hope and the faith to believe they are "more than conquerors through him who loved us" (Rom. 8:37 NIV). Hearing client testimonies of moms and dads *never* gets old! These tangible examples of people who were rescued from fear, found hope, and began to dream again are remarkable.

Adoption Unleashes Purpose

The real-life stories I hear through the work of our organization hit home with me. On the one hand, I know very well what it feels like to be pregnant in a less-than-ideal situation. I know the difficulties of single parenting. On the other hand, I know the blessing of being a parent who has found stability and is in a position to love and nurture a child whose biological parents were not equipped to do so. I have experienced the absolute joy that comes from loving and being loved by those whose birth mothers chose life for them. I have seen with my eyes that *adoption unleashes purpose.*

The reality is that my family of six would simply not exist without birth mothers who overcame adversity and viewed adoption as a viable path forward. My husband and best friend on the planet, Ryan, was blessed to have a courageous birth mom who chose to carry him for nine months through a traumatic pregnancy. Ryan was conceived in rape. Many people, including Christians, believe abortion is justified in cases of rape and incest—which comprise less than one percent of all abortions in America. But punishing with abortion those who have had no say over the circumstances surrounding their conception is not the answer. I rejoice that it wasn't the answer for Ryan's birth mother either. The world would assume that Ryan was "unwanted and unloved" based on his birth mom's heart-wrenching story. Yet her decision to reject abortion enabled his life to be seen as having equal and inherent value. She made a plan of adoption for Ryan and placed him into a family where the beauty of adoption is continually apparent.

Ryan's parents, after having three biological children, adopted ten others. Yes, you read that right. There were *thirteen* children in the Bomberger household. The family, albeit large—and when together resemble a United Nations gathering!—was very normal for all of them, and so was talking about adoption. Sitting around the table during holidays and hearing stories of "when mom and dad brought so-and-so home" was commonplace. Adoption wasn't something to be embarrassed about. It was simply one of the potential and beautiful results of a birth mother possessing the courage and conviction to choose life.

I am overcome with emotion whenever I reflect on the decision of Ryan's birth mom, as he says, "to give her son the gift of life *and* the gift of adoption." Her sacrifice and love have blessed me in ways she could have never thought possible. Because of her, I know the love of a phenomenal husband. Not only that, our four kiddos know the love of a father who is involved in the details of their lives and is actively creating a legacy with eternal ramifications. Ryan's life has had incalculable influence not only on me and our children but on countless people around the world. Through our foundation, Ryan speaks to and inspires hundreds of thousands of listeners each year, and he creates media content that empowers millions with the truth that life has purpose. His worth is not based on his accomplishments. We all have the same value simply because the Creator gives us worth. The decision of Ryan's birth mom was not only a gift to him but to all of us.

Ryan's birth story is not the only way that adoption has blessed my family. We continue to be one of many tangible examples of how the myth of the unwanted child is refuted over and over again. In 2006, Ryan and I were married just before my oldest daughter turned two. Our marriage came after I had chosen to leave an emotionally abusive relationship, one that resulted in my first pregnancy. My daughter's biological father did not want to be involved in our lives. Regardless of her biological father's refusal to parent, and despite all the fear that came along with parenting on my own, I chose life for her. For nearly two years, I was a single parent. Knowing that God had helped me walk away from an abusive situation, I worked tirelessly to create a life for my daughter that allowed God to be my main focus, strength, and source of wisdom. God's precious love (and my determination to stay out of the "crazies"), manifested in the gift of Ryan. He is a man who loves God deeply. From that deep well he loved me and my daughter with his whole heart. After years of custody battles and miracles that are so numerous they would fill a book all their own, her biological father voluntarily surrendered his parental rights. This allowed for the beautiful possibility of adoption to become a reality for my daughter and for Ryan, the man who was meant to be her father.

But that's not the end of our story. When my daughter was six years old, and our biological children were two and one respectively, the Lord connected us with a mom who was in the midst of a difficult season in life. We were able to walk alongside her and her older son as she faced an unplanned pregnancy. Despite the voices that were encouraging her to abort, she bravely opted to carry the pregnancy to term. Shortly after the Lord had our paths cross, she gave birth to the sweetest little boy. He had a number of medical challenges. Since we lived several states away, we were only able to pray and be a support system from afar. During this time, God sent her incredible family members to speak life and hope into her situation. In addition, they were able to care for the baby physically. The godly counsel his birth mom received during these weeks helped her to realize the beauty of giving her newborn son the gift of adoption. As a result, she bravely chose me and Ryan to adopt her son.

Although the circumstances surrounding these two adoptions were radically different, they both came with significant battles—some expected and many unexpected. Despite these challenges, we were ultimately faced with two options. Would we give up and walk away *or* press in deeper to our heavenly Father and believe for what seemed impossible? We learned repeatedly, both individually and together, to choose the latter—because there is *no such thing* as an unwanted child. Even if we feel rejected by those whom we think should be our support, every single human is wanted. Ryan and I knew the Lord had given us an opportunity to fight for these kids to show how much they are loved, valued, and belong in our family.

We learned, as a couple, to suit up with the armor of God. We delved deeply into the Word of God. It was typical to see Bible verses taped on the cabinet doors in the kitchen, on the bathroom mirrors, and even some attached to the dashboard of our car. Ryan and I were determined to commit to memorizing verses that gave us hope to combat moments of hopelessness. Scripture would help us replace doubt with powerful reminders of faith. We prayed and then prayed some more. Our friends would frequently get texts and emails with updates so they could be praying specifically for situations as they would arise. From a very young age we would have our children do the same. My oldest daughter's routine bedtime prayer was, *"Dear God, please thwart the plans of the enemy over my life. Thank you for the victory. Amen."* At times we would stay awake for hours and cry out to God, pleading for His intervention. As a result of battling hard, we have experienced many victories and, ultimately, finalizing the adoption of our oldest and youngest children. This spurs our faith on and helps us continue to encourage others to choose life, support those who are struggling with parenting, advocate for adoption, and defy the myth of the unwanted child.

Adoption—God's Plan

Embracing adoption should be a natural inclination for those who follow Christ. As Christians, we know there can be no salvation without adoption. Ephesians 1:4–5 says, "In love he predestined us for adoption to sonship through Jesus Christ, in accordance with his pleasure and will" (NIV). Our heavenly Father, through Christ, gives us the option to be adopted as His children. All we have to do is accept His offer and we become knit into His family forever. We take on His name, and His righteousness covers our unrighteousness. With such great love He allows us access to His nature, and we are grafted into His family. This deep and satisfying love and acceptance allows us the opportunity to find our identity in Him.

This is such a beautiful plan of redemption. So, of course, the enemy hates it! As Christians, we must expect that the ensuing spiritual conflict is inevitable. Knowing that adoption is warfare, we are less inclined to see the obstacles as a deterrent. We understand that we are warriors fighting for the souls of human beings created in the image of God. The enemy will never have the legacy that God's redeemed creation has as co-heirs with the King of kings (Rom. 8:17). Because of this truth, he is on a relentless mission to steal, kill, and destroy us at our most vulnerable moments. His jealousy and sheer hatred perpetuate his ruthless mission to see that precious image denied and erased.

As Christians, we cannot let the enemy win. Adoption is a part of a divine plan that transforms brokenness into wholeness, in the natural and supernatural. Yet so few Christians embrace this plan or understand the different roles we can all play in it.

Sadly, we are seeing the rates of adoption decline. According to the National Council for Adoption, the latest published study reported 110,373 total adoptions in the United States in 2014. Compare that with 175,000 in 1970 before *Roe v. Wade*. I believe a major factor in this decline is that the church, as a whole, neglects to place an emphasis on foster care and adoption. As Christians we should be leading the charge to adopt. James 1:27 defines "pure and genuine religion" as "caring for orphans and widows" (NLT). As of the middle of 2020, there were over 71,000 children eligible and waiting for adoption in our nation's foster care system.[6] If only one family in 17 percent of all Christian congregations would adopt a child, there would be no more children languishing in the system.[7] According to the Gospel Coalition, "If we divided all congregations into six groups, each group of churches would need to adopt one additional child every five years to ensure most all children always had a home. This is certainly within the realm of possibility."[8] Yes! This should be easily attainable.

However, it will never be a reality if Christians continue to remain uninformed and fearful of the adoption process. When Christians fail to act, children end up languishing in foster care or worse, aborted because it is believed that they are "unwanted." Souls that we could be shepherding and discipling for the kingdom are left as forgotten. This is why James 1:27 reminds us not to allow ourselves to be polluted by the world. The world promotes the myth of the "unwanted" child because they view poverty, adversity, and inequality as insurmountable challenges. But, as Christians with a biblical worldview, we see these hurdles as opportunities for our God to move on our behalf, teach us more about His victorious nature, and equip us to overcome.

Part of advocating well is engaging in conversations about the happy and hard parts of adoption. We have to talk about it all. We must confront the difficulties and celebrate the victories. As noted earlier, adoption is a means to help bring wholeness and healing. Where there is brokenness, there is struggle. But let's be real. We live in a broken world with fallen humanity. Regardless of our desire to steer clear of problems in life, there will *always* be tough situations to navigate. Parenting both adopted and biological children has proven to me that shepherding hearts will come with challenges regardless of the origin of the child. We embrace it all, as parents, because that's what we do! It's so upsetting to me when people close their hearts off to adoption because they believe the lie that the obstacles will be too great. I have heard it all. "There is too much trauma in adopting a kid." "Adoption is too expensive." "There is too much red tape." Ryan and I have seen the truth firsthand with each of these claims. Life is never devoid of difficulty, but love allows us to navigate, address, and usher healing where it is needed, no matter the circumstance. But are we called to live in fear of the unknown, or to walk in faith and see God work? He gives us hundreds of promises in the Bible, because humanity needs to be reminded *repeatedly* that "with God all things are possible" (Matt. 19:26 NIV).

Conclusion

We have what the world never will—true hope. Hope crushes the lie that God's people are unwanted and unloved. This, in fact, is why Jesus came to earth as a (humanly) unplanned baby. He chose to model for us the incredible purpose and importance of His creation at every single stage of life. Yet even as the Son of God, He lived a life marked by human rejection. Many couldn't understand His worth and refused to affirm their own. Jesus challenged this despairing point of view by being Hope and Love personified, caring for the marginalized and the magnified. It is up to us, as Christ's representatives, to carry these life-giving truths to a world that so desperately needs to understand its God-given worth. It is up to us to encourage moms and dads facing unplanned pregnancies to understand all things are possible.

Abortion is life-ending. Adoption is life-giving. It is up to us to lovingly illuminate the difference.

10

Mom, Thank You for Choosing Life: The Perspective of an Abortion Survivor

—Sarah Zagorski—

Redeem me from the oppression of man,
that I may keep Your precepts.
Psalm 119:134 NKJV

I can imagine my mother lying there on the table shaking, legs in stirrups, as she heard the words depart from the abortion doctor's lips: "Your daughter will be a mental vegetable incapable of having a normal life. You should leave her to die on the table." I can almost see her surroundings as she lay bare in front of the physician. Perhaps there were blood-stained linens beneath her, rusty medical equipment beside her, and maybe my tiny feet were just barely in her view.

I can imagine the fear my mom encountered as she realized,

suddenly, her life and precarious circumstances were colliding with the life of her own child, all while the physician pressed her for a response. She quickly mustered up the ten words that would save my life: "I'll sue you if you don't provide her medical care."

In January of 1990, infamous New Orleans abortion physician Dr. Ifeanyi Okpalobi had every intention of leaving me for dead following a breech delivery at 26 weeks' gestation. I was not breathing when I was born, so he determined I would be better off dead and that my family would be better off without me. My mother, Lidia, was initially referred to Dr. Okpalobi by a friend who convinced her that he helped poor immigrant women like herself by providing "cheap" services.

She courageously demanded that I receive appropriate medical care even though she knew she couldn't afford to care for and sustain the life of another child. She realized that neither she nor Dr. Okpalobi was qualified to make life-and-death decisions, to adjudicate permanent determinations about my future. She knew abortion was murder.

Now, I can imagine what could have happened if Lidia had given in to her fear and hadn't fought for my life, because I have spent years piecing together her story, my own close encounter with death, and learning about what happens behind closed doors at the hands of shoddy abortionists. (Dr. Okpalobi died in 2018.)

In 2013, the world learned more about the nature of late-term abortions following a premature delivery like mine, specifically from the criminal trial of former Philadelphia abortionist Dr. Kermit Gosnell. To ensure fetal demise following a live birth, Dr. Gosnell would "snip" the neck of newly born infants with scissors, severing their spinal cord.[1] A noteworthy commonality between my mother's physician and physicians like Dr. Gosnell was that they often attracted low-income clientele who would be less likely to report abuse or criminal medical practices.

It came to light, too, during Dr. Gosnell's trial that he performed abortions largely on minority women like my mother. And although Dr. Okpalobi of New Orleans didn't have Dr. Gosnell's record, his facility, Gentilly Medical Clinic for Women, had some of the same grotesque conditions. This clinic had previously been investigated by the Department of Health and had been shut down for a period of three years.[2]

Regardless of his mishaps, Dr. Okpalobi was the medical professional my mother turned to for help, and without her swift, brave action, my fate was sure. In the end, my mother fought for my survival. The abortion physician obliged, and I was sent to Children's Hospital's trauma birth ward in New Orleans. I believe Dr. Okpalobi was compelled to act only because he had been sued nine months earlier, in March 1989, for leaving the remains of a baby in a woman's uterus, making my mother's threat of legal action persuasive enough for him to provide me assistance.[3]

My mother's resistance saved my life. But while there is no doubt it was incredibly heroic, it was too much information for me to handle when I first learned about it as a young child in foster care. I held her choice to pursue abortion against her, thinking of myself as her judge and jury. I always glossed over the most important part of the story—that in the end, she chose rightly—she chose life.

Fear Leads to Abortion's Door

At first, my thinking about my mother's decision to fight for my life was clouded by my own hurt—hurt from her choice to pursue abortion in the first place, as well as the years of abuse and neglect

I experienced in her home prior to my adoption at the age of nine. Tragically, she passed away in 2010 when I was twenty years old, and I never had the opportunity to thank her for her pro-life decision. I could not understand the gravity of her suffering or the cruelty of her oppressors, but I certainly understand them now.

As a child, when I originally heard the story, I believed I was unwanted and that my mother tried to take the easy way out instead of carrying her pregnancy to term. It seemed pretty simple, and in the eyes of a young girl, sure, she saved me, but only after almost killing me. I knew there was never an excuse, never a justification for taking an innocent life, and at the time I didn't have the ears to hear more of my mother's story. If I had, I would have come to know that it was *oppression-driven fear* that led her to abortion's door, and her fear was well founded.

My mother was afraid my affluent, astute birth father would abandon her—*he did*. She was afraid her depression and mental illness would prevent her from providing for my basic needs—*it did*. She was afraid her sexually perverse husband and abusive sons would prey on me—*they did*. She was afraid that in the end she would lose me—*and she did*. Her fear was grounded in reality.

Don't worry, I am not going to announce now that my beliefs on abortion have evolved and I have "progressed" toward a shift in supporting abortion rights. I spend every day working with Louisiana Right to Life to make it unfathomable. And make no mistake, I look forward to the day *Roe v. Wade* is overturned. I know all too well that my mother's shattered heart couldn't be repaired by shattering the bones of her unborn children.

Yet my mother's torment was unrelenting, and her sorrow never diminished by dismembering her babies in abortion. In fact, the opposite is true. The two abortions she had prior to my conception only compounded her grief and furthered her mental anguish.

Thankfully, in recent years I have slowed down and taken time to survey her life. I have considered the complicated factors that lead women like her to commit the sin of killing their own children and have reflected on what we as Christians can do to prevent it. I believe I have come across an invaluable secret in my search in understanding abortion-vulnerable women and how we reach them before they end the life of their unborn child. A part of the way we end abortion actually resides in learning about the oppression-driven fear that leads them to that choice in the first place.

"Redeem me from the oppression of man, that I may keep Your precepts," David pleads with God following exile from his own country (Ps. 119:134 NKJV). Job curses the day he was born while being oppressed by Satan (see Job 3). And the writer of Ecclesiastes emphatically claims that the dead are more fortunate than those living under oppression. In fact, even more fortunate than the dead are those who never existed.

> I observed all the oppression that takes place under the sun. I saw the tears of the oppressed, with no one to comfort them. The oppressors have great power, and their victims are helpless. So I concluded that the dead are better off than the living. But most fortunate of all are those who are not yet born. For they have not seen all the evil that is done under the sun. (Eccl. 4:1–3 NLT)

Under cruel oppressors, humankind is tempted to do things it would ordinarily never consider, because oppression breeds fear. I watched this game ensue in my childhood as my mother attempted but ultimately failed to completely protect her children from the cycle of poverty, abusive family members, and the consequences of her own neglect. I discovered there that oppression bred fear, and sin frequently followed close behind.

In *The Treasury of David,* Baptist preacher Charles Spurgeon, commenting on Psalm 119:134, expounds on the link between oppression and sin. Spurgeon goes as far as to say that "to be oppressed is to be tempted," arguing that "we little know how much our virtue is due to our liberty." He explains, "He who taught us to pray, 'Lead us not into temptation,' will sanction this prayer, which is of much the same tenor, since to be oppressed is to be tempted."[4]

For my mother, oppression followed by fear was abortion's doorway, as it enticed her to act against her conscience. And oppression is the life theme of many abortion-minded women, of whom my mother was an archetype of sorts. My mother was just like the majority of women who have abortions, and she lived in constant fear.

An Archetype of the Abortion-Vulnerable Woman

My mother was economically disadvantaged, meaning she lived well below the Federal Poverty Level (FPL). Nearly 50 percent of women that had abortions in 2014 lived below the FPL, while 26 percent lived two times beneath it.[5] Simply stated, 75 percent of women who have abortions are poor, the kind of poor that leads to desperate choices.

My mother was a minority woman, too, a foreigner to America who learned English after she arrived in this country as a young teenager. According to the *American Journal of Public Health,* women like her (particularly Hispanic and African American women) account for the majority of abortions that take place in our country.[6] The abortion rate for Hispanic women is double that of White women, while the abortion rate for African American women is four times that of White women.[7] The truth is women of color are much more likely to abort, largely because they experience victimization on a larger scale than White women, and that correlates to their abortion vulnerability.

In 2015, 43 percent of all abortions in the United States were accounted for by women that already had one or two abortions, like my mother, and women that had more than three abortions accounted for eight percent.[8]

Additionally, my mother was a victim of domestic violence in her childhood and in her marriages, like many of the women who pursue abortion. She was born in Honduras, fled to America from an abusive father, and then became caught in the cycle of abusive marriages. Her first husband married her to gain US citizenship, and beat her on a regular basis. Her second was an abusive alcoholic who sexually molested her children. But my biological father weaponized his intelligence and privilege for his own gain. Women who abort "experience domestic violence and sexual assault up to three times the rate of those who continue with their pregnancies."[9] And statistically speaking, women in these circumstances are the women walking into abortion facilities.

In a lifetime, these factors are some of the puzzle pieces to my mother's life of sorrow, to her abortion vulnerability, and to the difficulties I witnessed in my own childhood. I did not have all her puzzle pieces then, but I have them today. These realities of her life, coupled with racial prejudice and economic inequality, came together to foster fear—just as they do for most abortion-minded women.

I have learned, too, that women like my mother are those whom Christ bids us to approach with a well of grace—a depth I just did not have in childhood, or even when my mother died in 2010. We must approach these women with grace combined with unwavering conviction that abortion will not solve their dilemmas. Abortion can't eradicate poverty, racism, or humankind's predatory tendency to hurt the vulnerable. Through Christ, though, Christians can help the vulnerable.

The Truth about "Unwanted" Children Like Me

It breaks my heart to say it, but the truth is I didn't have ears to hear my mother's story before her death. She made my life messy, and constant contact with her made my healing unattainable. She was the beaten traveler on the side of the road, and I was anything but her Good Samaritan. I regret that I was too focused on my own rescue story, on my own escape.

I, somehow, overlooked the part where, on encountering unbearable oppression, my mother turned from my mistaken villain to *hero*, by determining to make one of the most courageous decisions of her life: by choosing life rather than escaping fear. It is my belief that she'd had a recent encounter with Christ that brought about such heroic courage—heroic courage it took me years to see.

A deeper understanding of my mother's life helps me see today that her "unwanted pregnancy" had more to do with fear than with me as a person. I believe this is significant because many proponents of abortion argue that women should not have to raise unwanted children—children like me. They fail to recognize that in the majority of abortion cases, the child is not *truly* unwanted, and that if the mother's fears were stripped away, they would choose life for their baby.

My experiences with abortion-vulnerable women combined with statistical data about the hardships they face indicate that women choose abortion largely because of economic instability, abusive relationships, or racial prejudices that make them especially susceptible. After having to face the intimidating power of some men and of various other systems of inequality, these vulnerable women wrongly decide that abortion is their only choice. Fear has the final say in their pregnancy decision.

A quick glance at abortion statistics doesn't always give us the comprehensive picture and misleads some to the conclusion that women abort largely for the sake of convenience or because they genuinely don't want to raise their baby. There are definitely times when that is accurate, but a closer examination of the lives and circumstances of most women choosing abortion shows they are not killing their babies because they don't want their children. They are not killing their babies because they are thirsty for wealth, success, or any of the ungodliness that often first comes to mind. It is fear of their oppressors that leads them to abort.

I regret my own inability to have understood this as a child, but my one comfort is I know it was impossible for me to see through my mother's eyes back then, as her daughter, as one who suffered because of her decisions and negligence. She was a victimized woman, and I was a victim as a result. Since then, God has helped me forgive my mother and forgive myself for my lack of grace. He also enables me to be the Good Samaritan for other women in her shoes. Therein too I have found the redemption I could not see when she died, the redemption I could not fathom while burying her body in the ground.

Giving Thanks, Giving Grace

The truth is I would not be here if it were not for my mother's courage and obedience. My thank-you to my mother is long overdue.

> *Thank you, Mom, for choosing life and for leading me to the road that will help Christians bring about an end to abortion. I am just beginning to unearth all the ways God is redeeming your life. I know I wasn't unwanted by you; you were mistreated in a world that believed the lie that abortion was the only solution for your dilemmas.*

But beyond thanksgiving, certainly we have more to offer these women and their children because we know Jesus died to purchase their liberation—indeed, *my* liberation—from oppression-driven fear. Certainly, we know He's calling us to be His vessels by providing them with His solutions to social problems without compromising on abortion.

First, though, before the solution-finding, I urge you to do the hard, painstaking heart-work of rejecting the assumption that all or even most women walking into abortion facilities are villains. My mother was not my villain; she was a sinner no different from me, suffering under cruel oppressors. I can only pray I would have made the same heroic choice that she ultimately made by rejecting fear and choosing life.

For the Christ-follower, the unchanging truth that abortion is killing and a sin against God Himself is not up for debate. But our role is not to pass judgment but to respond with compassion, which should have been my response to my birth mother. Please learn from my mistake.

I am thankful we do not have to look far to find that it was actually Jesus' purpose in coming to earth to reach women like Lidia, and we don't have to wonder or hesitate in knowing what to do about the social problems that lead women to abort. In fact, a powerful verse sums it up: "*Learn* to do right; seek justice. Defend the oppressed. Take up the cause of the fatherless; plead the case of the widow" (Isa. 1:17 NIV, emphasis added).

The most compelling part of this verse to me is the prophet's use of "learn," for it indicates that study and practice are necessary to become proficient in seeking justice, and in my life, it is an art birthed in great pain. I am encouraged, however, that Isaiah is the one who later prophesies Jesus would be the Man of Sorrows (Isa. 53:3), whose victory over death would bring good news to the oppressed (Isa. 61:1–7). He is a Man of Sorrows who, if we take the time not only to study Him but to become like Him, will reveal His way to freedom from fear for the abortion-minded woman. I trust that He will reveal to you, too, that in order to become like Him, you must also slow down to learn about the suffering of the people He died to save.

Good News for You, Expecting Mother

If you are reading my story today and find yourself in my mother's shoes—or shoes like hers, where abortion appears to be your only option—please hear me out. I see you, and I know you may already carry the responsibilities of motherhood. Are you running from an abusive relationship? Are you unsure of where the next few meals will come from? Are your other children already suffering behind the four walls of your home? I know your fear because I also lived pinned down by the weight of those difficulties. My own eyes have seen the unspeakable darkness behind those walls.

Today, too, I can imagine you walking into that abortion facility feeling hopeless and paralyzed by those circumstances. I can almost hear your trembling voice as you talk to the receptionist. I can envision your despair as you take your seat next to the other women wrestling through similar nightmares. *But please wait; please don't kill your baby, because I have good news for you, expecting mother. I have hope to offer you.* You see, by God's grace I lived to see the world outside of oppressive walls. I *lived* to see humanity at its best because my mother lassoed the fear in her heart, the fear you are encountering right now.

She lassoed fear by rejecting abortion and giving me the opportunity to escape. The depravity of my childhood home did not destroy me. My mother's oppressors didn't get the last word, and her mistakes as a mother did not have final authority over my life. I escaped death's grasp because of her courage, and I found that on the other side many pro-life people were waiting to help me and my family.

Take that first step and walk toward life.

CLAIM 5

My Circumstances Justify Ending My Pregnancy

11

Embracing Life's Bump: Experiencing God's Grace in Teenage Pregnancy

—Amy Ford—

Right before my teenage years came to a close, at nineteen years old, I found myself with an unexpected pregnancy. Even though I grew up in church, I didn't have a close relationship with the Lord. I loved my boyfriend very much, but we had begun looking to each other for validation, instead of to God.

I had also grown up thinking abortion was wrong, but once I saw that positive pregnancy test, abortion became a real option for me. Fear had taken over and consumed all my thinking. I convinced myself that an abortion would be the easiest way out. Ryan and I would never have to tell a soul; we would never have to disappoint our families. We could deal with a broken heart later, but we felt an urgency to make our "bump in life" go away.

I went about for a few weeks in a robotic-like state, just trying not to feel. My brain still had a hard time processing what was going on. I would try to picture myself as a young mom, but I really couldn't see it. I couldn't see past even telling my parents. I was so worried about disappointing my family. All the worst-case scenarios went through my head—being the black sheep of the family, my parents hating me, getting kicked out of the house and being homeless. Every thought I had was rooted in fear. I felt as if I had no one to reach out to because I knew I would be letting down my family and friends.

Ryan did some research and found an abortion clinic in our city. We set our appointment and paid the fee. I came within moments of having an abortion, having made it as far as being in a medical gown and sitting on the cold table. While the nurses were describing how they would perform the abortion and what was about to happen, all the emotions I had tried so hard not to feel suddenly overpowered me. I had an anxiety attack, hyperventilated, and passed out.

Then, as the nurses were fanning me and trying to get some water into my system, one of them looked me in the eyes and said, "You're too emotionally distraught to make this decision today. You can come back another day, but today you're not getting an abortion." I walked back to the waiting room. Ryan saw that my eyes were red and my face was swollen from crying. "We're still pregnant," I told him.

Deep down I knew that having this abortion would affect me for the rest of my life. In that moment, we decided just to see what would happen if we *chose life*. We would take whatever consequences that awaited us. We were nervous about our future and about how our families would respond to the news. But we became determined to figure it out together and to brace ourselves for the hard months ahead.

Ryan and I married when I was sixteen weeks pregnant. The first pastor that we asked to marry us said that he couldn't officiate the wedding or bless the marriage because we had sinned. One by one, friends left. Looking back, I know it wasn't because they no longer liked me—they just didn't know what to do or say. Our pregnancy was the "elephant in the room." People didn't know whether to say "Congratulations," or "I'm sorry," so they didn't say anything at all.

Before getting pregnant I had been active in the church and had a lot of friends there. After getting pregnant, I tried going back to church, but things had changed. No one acknowledged the pregnancy and the baby growing inside me. It was as if they couldn't see me. For some, it was hard to make eye contact. I felt invisible. So I left, and stayed away for many years.

I eventually returned to the church and raised my son to love the Lord. Jess is now twenty-one years old. He has received a degree in theology from Oral Roberts University and recently married Audrey, the love of his life. It's unbearable to think about what life would look like without him. He has led many kids to the Lord and has a passion for evangelism. Knowing his story has helped him understand all the more that God has a plan for his life. Jess says, "I was an overcomer before I was even born. Satan had a plan to take me out. But I'm here and I'm going to use my life however the Lord wants to use me."

Still, going through an unplanned pregnancy at a young age was very difficult. We were so close to losing our precious son because of fear. Because of isolation. Because of shame and feeling that there was no one who would understand. And our experience is not unique. My heart breaks for every teenage momma considering abortion, knowing all the emotions overwhelming her. I know what I needed most during that season was community, a place of belonging where I could open up without fear of being judged or shamed.

Facing the Fear of Teen Pregnancy

My experience has fueled my passion for young women going through similar circumstances, while also having an impact on how I go about trying to help them. I no longer speak about the abortion debate as I did before. My thoughts haven't changed; I still know it is wrong. But now instead of talking about abortion dogmatically, I address the issue with compassion and empathy, meeting women where they are in their place of fear.

There may be different reasons behind every woman's choice, but all of them are rooted in fear. My friend Destiny, who had an unplanned pregnancy as a teen, said it best, and gave me permission to share her words:

> See, you don't realize how temporary the "crisis" is when it's consuming your every waking moment, but as soon as you get beyond that . . . such beauty can be born from that which we never planned. Fear is temporary, but the courage you gain facing it lasts forever. Panic subsides, but the strength you find in the midst of the crisis endures. Perhaps the most amazing thing though is how the love you feel for this new life, whether it was intended or not, suddenly turns a "mistake" into a miracle. I didn't save my son by "choosing life." He saved me.

Girls like Destiny should not have to face an unplanned pregnancy alone. We all have something to offer young moms that can help empower them. The recipe for transforming fear to faith is simple. There is just one ingredient—love. "Perfect love drives out fear" (1 John 4:18 NIV). Love saves lives.

We can't just vote a certain way or talk about what needs to change. We *are* the change. And it will take all of us to create change. There are so many ways that people are helping and loving teen moms practically. But many people who want to help do not feel equipped or know about the awesome resources that are out there.

I used to feel the same way. A few years ago, I didn't even know there was a pro-life movement or organizations whose purpose it was to help women with unplanned pregnancies. After the release of my first book, *A Bump in Life*,[1] I received invitations to speak for various organizations. One of them was a Care Net Conference, a training conference for pregnancy center workers. When I arrived at the conference, there were hundreds of pro-life ministries lining the hotel hallways to share information about a service or life-saving ministry that people could connect and get involved with. I walked up and down those halls in awe of how many amazing services were available. I kept thinking, *If only people knew about all these resources!*

The pro-life movement is filled with love and empowerment. There are organizations that are already doing great things, and there are people who help individually, using the strengths, gifts, and passions God put inside of them to make a difference. And it's important that they do help. Approximately 550,000 pregnancies occur annually among teen women ages 15 to 19 years old in the United States.[2] Whether teen moms choose to parent or choose to place their baby for adoption, they will need a lot of practical help as well as emotional support along the way. Let me provide a few tips for how Christians can come alongside pregnant teenage moms.

Pregnancy and Parenting Support

Experiencing an unplanned pregnancy can be completely overwhelming to a teenage single mom. And navigating motherhood after the baby has arrived can be even more overwhelming. It isn't easy figuring out day care, finding and keeping a job that will provide enough income, working with the school to adjust classes around the delivery, establishing co-parenting routines with the baby's father (if he's even involved), and much more. The teen mom needs all the assistance she can receive.

Having a strong and healthy family support system, one that allows the mom to raise her child in the family home until she can get on her feet, is always the best and easiest option for her. She needs extra support so she can focus on finishing school and working to pay her bills. For moms who do not have a supportive family system and find themselves homeless during pregnancy, maternity homes are located throughout the United States that provide housing and allow a single and pregnant mom time to catch her breath, receive healing, make a game plan for income, and work on job security. It is absolutely free for the mom in need and can be the launching pad for her next season of being a young mom. I have also seen members of churches open their homes to both single pregnant moms and single young moms while they focus on their education and on raising their child. A stable home environment is critical for a young mom to flourish.

If a pregnant teen is in high school, it can be a challenge, but it is possible to have a child and still graduate. There's no way to sugarcoat it. There will be obstacles along the way, like possible morning sickness that makes it hard to get up for school, or regular doctor visits that may result in frequent absenteeism. Also, it's just hard to be in high school when you are pregnant because of social stigmas. High schoolers can be hurtful and rude; the stares and comments are not easy to ignore. But having supportive friends who cheer the mom on along the way is what will keep them focused and determined. I know, for myself, it wasn't the person that I believed in the most who made the biggest difference in my life, it was the person who believed in *me*. And that's what teen mothers need—someone to believe in them.

Every teen mom has the right to go to school without being turned away because of pregnancy. The legal guide titled *Public Schools and Pregnant and Parenting Adolescents* says, "The [North Carolina] state constitution guarantees a right to education and promises equal opportunities for all students in the public schools."[3] This holds true in all states. Some schools even have counselors and nurses who will help guide the student as well as provide a parenting class at the school to help single young moms.[4]

Child care costs are also something that a teen pregnant mom may be concerned about. Child care can sometimes cost more than monthly food allowance, tuition, rent, or transportation. For many teen moms, assistance is available. Each state receives funds from the federal government for a state-run child care subsidy program. These programs help low-income families pay for child care so they can work or attend school. Eligibility requirements are different in each state.[5]

Roughly half of the colleges in the United States offer some type of child care. Having reliable and accessible child care on campus can help ensure a young mom finishes her degree and feels confident that her child is being cared for and close by.[6]

A pregnancy resource center is a great place for a teen mom to get help during the pregnancy and during the first few years of being a new mom. These centers are a jackpot of information in the community that can connect her to all the resources available. I've seen pregnancy centers give information about programs for child care subsidy, health care support, housing and maternity homes, as well as job information, to name just a few. Many give out free diapers and wipes, or have boutiques with gently used baby items for mommas in need.

Teen moms can also go through an Embrace Grace group at a local church. Embrace Grace is an international, church-based ministry I launched in 2012 in order to provide moms with the same emotional and material support I needed when pregnant with Jess. Located in over 700 churches, 47 states, and 10 countries, Embrace Grace is a 12-week support group that will empower a mom facing an unplanned pregnancy to be brave and choose life. The group provides her with a spiritual family and community within the church, as well as with a baby shower providing all the baby items needed—and all brand new! We want the church to be one of the first places a girl runs to, instead of the last, when she faces an unexpected pregnancy. And we want these moms to raise their kids in the church and get involved. When a new mom knows she is not alone, she feels a renewed peace of mind. She might not have everything figured out, but she can relax, knowing there are people and programs that will help along the way. And the church is a great place to find people who are willing to help.

I remember the first group that I ever led. One mom wore a coat in August, in Texas, because she was terrified of stepping foot inside the church and for anyone to see her growing tummy. By the end of the semester, she had completely changed. She was empowered, as a woman and as a mother, to be the mom that God created her to be. She was transformed from the inside out.

Having now helped churches around the world open their doors and hearts to women experiencing unexpected pregnancies, I have seen how strong family support, whether coming from a spiritual family or a biological family, plays a huge role in how a teen mom will not only survive but thrive as she embarks on motherhood at such a young age.

Adoption Support

I've had a lot of conversations with teen moms who are thinking about having an abortion, and when I bring up the option of adoption, they immediately shut it down. I ask them why, and for the most part they say, "I don't know. That would just be weird. I can't give my baby away."

Twenty-plus years ago, adoption was a lot less popular than it is today. There was a lot of shame surrounding adoption, with some moms being sent away for an extended period of time so that their inner circle of family and friends would never have to know. Now the adoption discussion is more transparent in our society, especially because the number of open (as opposed to closed) adoptions has increased tremendously. Even so, we still have a lot of work to do to change birth moms' perception of adoption.

Adoption isn't an easy decision or process. It comes with an aftershock of heartache. Birth moms feel isolated and lonely immediately after they have released their baby into another family's care. Some feel much like a mother who experiences losing an infant or a pregnancy; there is an element of grief involved. What a birth mom needs most is someone to support her before, during, and after the process.

One of the main reasons a girl might choose adoption is because she faces financial hardship and may not be able to provide the life she wishes for her child. It's always good to start an imaginative conversation about what it would look like for her to have everything she needed. Encourage her to explore the possibilities and dream out loud. What would she need financially? Would she need a better job? Would she need a car? Would she need child care? Sometimes with a little help from a community of people, she can get the hand-up she needs to be able to parent her child.

If she wants to place her baby for adoption even after a conversation like this, there are many adoption agencies around the United States, some even that provide housing for the mom during the pregnancy and for an extended time after birth. Adoption can give pregnant women the power to make a plan and choose in the best interest of both herself and the baby. A birth mom can be matched with a great family she chooses, then meet and talk with them, getting to know them on a personal level. Open adoptions are very common, where the adoptive family corresponds through letters and pictures, so the birth mom can watch her child grow. Agencies cover most costs associated with the pregnancy and birth, and they help set the mom up for her next season after pregnancy.

It is always a joy to hear how birth moms find their adoptive families. Their adoption stories have a way of revealing how God has taken them on an adventure, sealing His words with amazing confirmations, and showing everyone involved that this is part of His plan.

I once worked with a mom who placed her son for adoption four years before. When she got married in a beautiful ceremony, her son had the joy and honor of being the ring-bearer in the wedding. It was a sweet scene. Another teen mom who placed her baby for adoption meets her daughter throughout the year on scheduled dates; the little girl even calls the birth mom her "Birthday Mom." The way

God connects the birth moms to the adoptive moms is always such a beautiful miracle. God tends to provide evidence of His fingerprints throughout the adoption process to give a birth mother courage and confirmation that she's making a good decision.

In a day when it is socially acceptable to end a pregnancy out of convenience, adoption stories are a breath of fresh air. These women have chosen to give life to their child. They are brave, courageous, and should be honored. The sacrifice is great, but the reward is greater.

Sarah's Story

In *A Bump in Life,* I shared a story about Sarah.[7] Sarah was nineteen, pregnant by a guy she never really knew and didn't even like very much. She was in a band and often drank, smoked pot, and stayed out late; she struggled with an eating disorder; and basically, Sarah was very unhappy. One day she told us the story about when she first found out she was pregnant.

Sarah had begun to suspect something was off, so she bought a pregnancy test and took it in her dad's bathroom. She couldn't believe it when she read the word "pregnant" on that little white stick. Her heart sank as a huge mix of crazy thoughts and emotions swirled inside of her.

There was no thinking about it—she could never raise a child—she was too young. She had never even changed a diaper! She had no idea how to be a parent! She knew abortion was her only option. But she also had no idea how she was going to manage scraping the money together to have the abortion.

Sarah spent weeks searching online for information on the procedure and any kind of financial assistance that might be available.

The more time she spent thinking, searching, and stressing, the more real the pregnancy felt. Her heart sank a little further as each day passed; she needed to make a decision quickly. First, she tried to explain herself to the baby. One night at Embrace Grace class, she said to us:

> I knew I might see her in heaven one day, and I didn't want her to think that I was being selfish (which, really, I was) or that I disliked her. I needed some time by myself to get control of my thoughts. I went to a horrible Mexican restaurant and took with me a pen, paper, and enough money to buy queso dip (that baby always wanted cheese). I sat down to write and stared at the paper blankly for fifteen minutes, just trying to keep my composure and not cry.
>
> I had so many confusing emotions. I kept thinking, *I have to do this. Anyone in my situation wouldn't have the baby either. There is no other way. I have way too many things going on in my life, and plus, I would be a terrible mother. I will lose everything in my life if I have this baby. The baby will be better off not being born to someone like me who can't even love a person. I can't love anyone. Look at the things I've done.*
>
> I took a deep breath and grabbed my pen. As I was holding it, those thoughts still echoed in my head: *baby . . . the baby, the baby,* over and over again. I couldn't think of *it* as a *baby,* or I would never be able to get rid of it and get my life back. I started writing.
>
> *Dear baby, I want you to know why I have to do this. I can't give you the love or the life that you need. I'm not ready to be a mom. I know you'll go to heaven because you're innocent and you'll be very happy there. Love . . .*

I was stuck. I didn't know how to sign it.

After I began to sign the letter with the word *love* at the end, I just froze. I couldn't sign it *"Love, Mom."* It hurt too much even thinking the word *Mom* knowing what I was about to do. I finally just quickly signed it *Me.* I folded it up and put it in my pocket.

I did this all to try to make myself feel better, but somehow, I left feeling much worse.

When I got home, I told my mom that I was pregnant and needed help. She did not want me to have an abortion and said she wouldn't help me do that. But she would help me keep the baby. I told my dad and I asked him if he still loved me, and he said that he did. But he couldn't even look at me for three weeks.

After weeks of thinking she needed to get an abortion but never actually going through with it, Sarah decided to keep her baby.

When word got out, most of her friends walked away, one by one. Her band even kicked her out—via text message—when they realized a pregnant lead singer wouldn't really give them the image they were trying to portray.

But there were beautiful moments too.

During her pregnancy, Sarah and her mother bonded like never before. For once, neither of them was selfish or self-absorbed, and everything they did was for the baby. Even though the father of the baby had walked out, Sarah began dating a guy who surprised her with ice cream every night. Never in her life had she felt so full and so free, all at the same time.

When Sarah was sharing her story at our Embrace Grace class, she started to cry, which was rare for her, as God began to reveal

Himself to her. She had known for a long time that God had been giving her some tough love, and she knew He wanted her to stop the lifestyle she had been living. She knew God was saying, "No more of this. No more self-destruction."

Since Sarah had difficulty making friends and nurturing relationships with people, even though she wanted them, she asked God to send an angel into her life so she wouldn't be alone.

That particular day in our class, while processing where her life had been and where her life was now going, she had the realization that this little girl she was carrying was the answer to those prayers. With eyes full of happy tears, she told us, "When I feel lonely, I just sing to her or just talk to her. Her little kicks and squirms feel like hugs and kisses. I can see that the world isn't this dark, unforgiving, harsh place that I thought it was—and I never want my daughter to view the world that way either. What I thought was punishment turned out to be God's greatest gift to me, and I was so undeserving. I used to cry and ask God, 'What did I do to deserve this?' Now I just wonder what I did to deserve this—this beautiful gift of life."

Sarah's life changed forever that day her beautiful baby was born. Nothing anyone said even mattered anymore, because now her little girl was right there in her arms. It was real. Her baby, whom she named Fiona, was perfect.

A few months after the baby was born, I spent some time mentoring Sarah and hanging out with her; I enjoyed her company a lot. She was like this unique treasure box, and every time I spent time with her, I would uncover more and more precious jewels inside of her.

One day she shared with me, "My life switched upside-down like crazy after my baby was born. It didn't totally happen all at once, though. It took a while for me to realize that my daughter was going to need all of me. She made me want to be a better person. God lit a little fire under me, and her name is Fiona."

> Since the day she was born, I've still made dumb mistakes. I always will, since I'm human. But God's presence in her is so clear to me. I still see with those new eyes He gave me in her. Every day a little bit more of her individuality is expressed and every day she brightens my life more and more. She reminds me to pray. She tells me, "Don't give up, Mama. It's okay. Try again. You can do it!" Every decision I make now is made based on wanting a better life for the two of us.
>
> From the time we are young and able to think, we have big dreams of changing the world, becoming something, impacting someone's life, or just doing something everyone will see as extraordinary. A child doesn't change that, doesn't slow the momentum. Your child is the change the world needs; your child is what makes you something. You'll impact his/her life beyond measure, and becoming a mother is one of the most extraordinary things you can do here on earth.

Sarah went on to finish her education and is now a nurse. Her baby was the fuel she needed to break away from toxic patterns and work toward her goals and future.

With a good support system and with advocates helping along the way, teen moms will feel braver and more empowered to choose life. Together, we can help her know that she can have her baby and her dreams too.

12

Hope Is Found in Hard Places: Pregnant during Financial Hardship

—Christina Bennett—

When I was in my twenties, my mom revealed a secret to me that she'd kept hidden all of my life. "You'll hate me if I tell you," she warned me. Months prior a woman at church approached me to say God told her something remarkable had happened around the time of my birth. I asked my mother, Andrea, and she told me she met an angel before I was born. She refused to talk about it further or answer any questions.

One summer, after arriving home from a ministry trip, I decided to ask my mom for the whole story. I approached her while she was getting ready for the day. After assuring her I would love her regardless of what she told me, she shared a secret that changed my life.

My mother revealed that while pregnant with me she made an appointment for an abortion at Mount Sinai Hospital in Hartford, Connecticut. In her heart she wanted me, but she was frightened by difficult circumstances. My parents were unmarried, and my father already had two children and didn't want another. He pushed her to have an abortion and she succumbed to that pressure.

My mom had a mentor at church she respected. She worked up the courage to confide in her about the pregnancy. To her great dismay, her mentor rejected her after learning she was having sex outside of marriage. "If you come back to this church, I will be the first person to put my foot in the door and not let you in," she said coldly. Feeling pressured, alone, and rejected, my mom made that appointment to abort.

Maybe you can relate to those feelings. You know what it is like to be faced with fears involving an unplanned pregnancy and overwhelming pressures. I want you to know you are not alone. I pray you find strength and encouragement in my mother's story.

Andrea's Story

Andrea was in her late twenties when she became pregnant with me. Her relationship with my father, Gerald, was less than ideal. Being unmarried and pregnant didn't carry the same stigma in the 1980s as it had decades earlier. Nevertheless, being single with an unplanned pregnancy wasn't in her game plan.

My mother and father are both Black, which ties them to the struggles our people group have faced for generations. Abortion isn't something we talked about in my family. Growing up, I didn't know the devastating impact abortion had on the Black community. Did you know Black women have been targeted by an abortion industry that is rooted in eugenics philosophy and a population control agenda? The film MAAFA21 on YouTube goes into great detail concerning this.[1] It is a sad truth I discovered later than I should have. With over 78 percent of abortion clinics in lower income and minority neighborhoods, Black women are five times more likely to abort than White women. Black women make up 14 percent of the childbearing population but account for 36 percent of all abortions.

It is not that Black women love their children any less than women of other races. It is not that women like myself and my mom are less capable of being great mothers. Tragically, women of color have been targeted by a greedy industry that financially profits from our painful circumstances. My mother told me the counselor she met at the hospital didn't give her options, advice, or good counsel. She was put in a medical gown as the counselor assured her, "You're making the best decision." Deep down my mother doubted those words.

In the darkest moments, God's light still shines. God can break into a seemingly hopeless situation, bringing His power and hope. It is remarkable how our lives can change drastically in a moment. The words from a stranger—whether in person, online, or in the pages of a book—can be exactly what we need to go forward. The counselor told my mom to go to the waiting room until the doctor called her name. Between the counselor's office and the waiting room was a hallway. She stopped for a moment to cry before her procedure. As she sat in the hallway with her head down, an elderly Black woman approached her. The woman was a janitor in the hospital. She walked up to my mom, lifted up her chin, and looked her in the eyes. "Do you want to have this baby?" she asked. Even though my mom already paid for the abortion, she said, "Yes." The woman said, "God will give you the strength to have this baby." The janitor's eyes were like pools of water. My mother felt peace just looking into them. The kind stranger told my mom to go back into the waiting room and get her clothes. As she walked away, my mom looked down for a few seconds to compose herself. Then she looked up, expecting to see the kind woman midway down the hallway with her mop and equipment. Instead, to my mom's surprise, she was gone.

My mother walked into the abortion doctor's office and saw blood on the floor. He hadn't even cleaned up from the last abortion appointment. Disgusted, she told the doctor she changed her mind and was leaving. At first the doctor responded by trying to calm her down. "You're just nervous," he said. She repeated that she had changed her mind and wanted to keep me. The doctor urged her to go through with the abortion. "You've already paid for it," he reminded her. My mother was firm. She wanted to leave. At this point the doctor got visibly angry. He raised his voice and yelled, "Don't leave this room!" Even though my mother was frightened, she refused to listen. She ran out of his office, called my dad on the lobby pay phone, and told him she didn't go through with the abortion.

My mom did not plan to tell me I was almost aborted. If a stranger at church hadn't said something "remarkable" had happened, I would never have known God rescued me minutes before a scheduled death. God longed for me to know how much He truly wanted me. He wanted me to know how brave and courageous my mother was in that terrifying moment. God was the one who sent that janitor to speak the words that saved my life. God never saw me as just a "choice"; He saw me as His beloved daughter.

Over time I have come to believe there is no such thing as an "unwanted child." The fear of an unplanned pregnancy causes some parents to end their child's life through abortion. Even in those situations, there may have been a family member who would have parented that child. If not in the family, someone in their church or community could have adopted the baby. As a foster and adoptive parent, I know there are thousands like me who choose to open their homes to children in need.

Circumstances Don't Define Us

Children are never less valuable because of the circumstances they are born into. Do you know many of the great leaders in history were survivors of difficult circumstances? Maya Angelou (1928–2014) was one of the most prolific Black female writers in our nation. As a child she suffered a sexual assault that left her speechless for years. She went from refusing to talk for a period of time in her youth to speaking before American presidents and world leaders in her elder years.

Harriet Tubman (c. 1822–1913) is well-known as a former slave and freedom fighter. She suffered a devastating head injury at the hands of a slave owner that gave her a life-long struggle with narcolepsy, seizures, and headaches. Yet her injury did not prevent her from rescuing hundreds of people from the chains of bondage.

Fannie Lou Hamer (1917–1977) was a civil rights activist who was born to poor sharecroppers in the South. She was the youngest of twenty children. Fannie was a smart girl, but she had to quit school at the age of twelve to pick cotton with her family. Fannie's family often went hungry, but she didn't let suffering stop her from pursuing her dreams. She became involved with civil rights work and organized voter drives. She helped countless African American young people register to vote in her home state of Mississippi. In 1961 Fannie was a victim of forced sterilization. A doctor was supposed to remove a uterine tumor but gave her a hysterectomy instead. That horrible experience led her to speak out against forced sterilization and abortion, which she called "a means of genocide of Blacks." Fannie and her husband could not have biological children, but they adopted two daughters. One of her favorite songs to sing was "This Little Light of Mine." Even though she suffered dark times, God's light shone through her.

Moses was a chosen deliverer whom God raised up to set the Israelites free from the cruelty of slavery. As a child, Moses's life was in danger of death. Out of fear of the Hebrews' population growth, Pharaoh ordered midwives to kill the males they helped birth. Thankfully, the Hebrew midwives chose to obey God over the command of Pharaoh. Moses's mother, Jochebed, saw that he was a beautiful child, and she hid him. She put him in a basket that was found by Pharaoh's daughter. Moses could have died as a baby, but instead he was adopted by royalty. His birth mother's courage allowed him to become a leader that set his people free from slavery.

Mary the mother of Jesus is another example of someone who, despite difficult circumstances, obeyed the call of God on her life. Mary was visited by the angel Gabriel who told her she had found favor with God and would give birth to a holy child by the power of the Most High. One can only imagine how frightened and confused Mary must have felt in that moment. She was young, not yet married, and chosen to birth the Savior and Messiah of the world. If that's not a description of being under pressure, I'm not sure what is! Yet even in the midst of Mary's complicated emotions, she surrendered herself to God, saying "Let it be to me according to your word" (Luke 1:38). Mary said yes to God, even when it didn't make sense.

The difficult circumstances surrounding these leaders didn't cause them to be worth any less as people, or to be any less useful in God's hands. Their challenges actually shaped them to become the leaders God called them to be. That's just how God uses our suffering and the trials we face—to grow us into people ready to be used by Him (Rom. 8:28–29; James 1:2–4).

God Provides

You may be in a situation like my mother was. You may want to keep your baby, but you are unsure how it will work. Perhaps it doesn't seem like the right time to have a child. I want you to know that there is never a perfect time to have a baby. As I write this, my husband and I have adjusted our lives to work from home for the past nine months. The global pandemic that came in the early months of 2020 changed our circumstances as it did for countless others. I never imagined an unexpected pandemic would take the lives of hundreds of thousands of Americans, and millions of people worldwide. Tens of millions of others throughout the world have lost jobs, housing, and loved ones.

The circumstances of this year revealed to me that the things I depend on for stability and security can be gone in a moment. At the same time, I have experienced breakthroughs and long-awaited answers to prayer. In the midst of the challenges of this year, I was blessed with a newborn baby whom I'm fostering on his way to adoption. While the arrival of this precious baby came during a time of unexpected difficulties, his presence is an answer to years of prayer.

Every day is full of unlimited potential and possibility. When one door closes, another door can open for you. Don't think that you can't have a baby just because you are lacking some kind of necessity. Be honest about your needs and what is causing you to fear parenting. Always know that God is a Provider who can and will meet your needs as you trust in Him. Your needs and desires always matter to God.

Along with being a Provider, God is also the Creator and giver of life. Psalm 139:13–14 says, "For you created my inmost being; you knit me together in my mother's womb. I praise you because

I am fearfully and wonderfully made; your works are wonderful, I know that full well" (NIV). God is the one who knits us together while we are in our mother's womb. God knows all His plans for us before we are even born.

The Truth about Abortion

I was born eight years after the Supreme Court decision *Roe v. Wade* legalized abortion. I never had an adult in my family or church talk to me about abortion as I was growing up. I heard abortion talked about in school as simply a women's right. Children in the womb were discussed as merely "clumps of tissue" or "lumps of cells" in society. I did not realize until adulthood that a baby's heartbeat starts at just five to six weeks. I did not know her lungs develop at eight weeks and she can kick by eleven weeks. When I was in high school, I lacked access to the internet. Social media didn't become so accessible until I was in college. Young people today have a wealth of information and knowledge at their fingertips. All you have to do is search "fetal development" on the internet to see the amazing wonder of life in the womb. Psalm 139:14 says we are "fearfully and wonderfully made," and you can see that "wonder" when you look at the development of a growing baby. Take a moment to look online at images of children in the womb. If God can knit a baby together in the womb, He can provide for their needs once they are born.

You may have been told that your challenging circumstances justify abortion. You might have heard that abortion is the responsible or right thing to do. Do you ever wonder how we got to a place where abortion is discussed as an acceptable option? Before 1973, the majority of people in our nation saw abortion as an unthinkable act. When the laws changed, public opinion soon followed. That is because the laws of our land shape the way we understand morality. When something is illegal, we grow up assuming that it is morally wrong. When something is legal, we believe that it is morally permissible. Maybe you were taught abortion is morally acceptable. Perhaps you were taught that it is just a choice a woman makes with her doctor. I can relate to that, as the truth of abortion was hidden from me for most of my life. I want you to know that ending the life of your baby is not a healthcare decision. The idea that having an abortion is just another medical procedure could not be further from the truth. Financial difficulties or hardships do not warrant ending your child's life.

A successful abortion always destroys the life of a unique, growing baby. Abortion is an act that hurts everyone involved. God is certainly a forgiving, merciful God, though having an abortion is making a choice that is irreversible. Many women who have had abortions come to God with their guilt, shame, and pain. Many have experienced forgiveness and healing after confessing their sins and accepting His love. Although they are grateful for healing, many regret the permanent decision they made to end their child's life. If they could go back and change things, they would. I know this because while working as a client services manager for a pregnancy center, I was able to sit and speak with women who had abortions. I have seen their pain and have become familiar with the regret that can come from choosing abortion.

I know women who had fetal remains left inside of them after an abortion. I know women who were left infertile and those who wrestled with suicidal thoughts. I have talked with women who mourn their aborted child's due date each year, thinking about how old they would now be if still alive. The emotional pain and trauma that comes from abortion can last a lifetime. I will never forget the gray-haired women who have approached me with tears in their eyes. I will never forget the hurting men. They have come up to me at events where I have spoken about abortion. They want me to know their stories and the pain abortion caused them. They know they are forgiven and loved by God, but the memory of a life lost remains with them.

Overcoming Unique Financial Challenges

You may be struggling with financial difficulties and wondering how you will afford a child. You may be unsure as to how you will pay your bills or get out of debt. I have met with many mothers who are dealing with similar hard circumstances, and I want you to know that even when things seem bleak, there is always hope.

I have seen mothers who were struggling to find a job gain good employment. I have helped mothers who were homeless find housing—some went to temporary shelters and maternity homes before getting their own places to live. I have aided pregnant women who struggled to work and who needed government assistance to pay for day care. I know women who went back to get their high school diploma or obtained their driver's license later in life. I know mothers and fathers who had to reach out to their extended family, friends, and church community to get the resources they needed to parent. There is no shame in reaching out for help.

It is hard to struggle and not to have your needs met. But you must remember that even in the hardest moments, life is still a beautiful gift worth fighting for. As human beings we are only given one life to live on this earth—and some of us will be born into riches and others into poverty. Some of us are born strong and healthy, while others are born with sickness and physical challenges. Some are born in war-torn lands and others are born in places of prosperity and freedom. It is easy to compare our lives to others. Scrolling through social media can cause our hearts to be filled with envy and anger, because there is always someone who has more than we do. And many who have less.

My mother raised my brother and me as a hard-working, single mom. She married my father after choosing not to abort me, but sadly, they divorced a year later. We struggled growing up as our mom tried her best, working as a secretary. We moved so often that I spent first grade to fifth grade in a different school every year. But in spite of the difficulties we faced, I knew I was loved by my mother, and that made all the difference. Yes, at times I envied the clothes and possessions of my cousins and friends who had more than I did; it is normal to struggle with wanting more. Yet throughout my entire life, even when I suffered lack, the Lord supernaturally provided for me. There has never been a time when God has not come through for me as a Father and Provider.

When I became an adult, I traveled to developing countries and saw poverty unlike anything I had ever experienced. I rode trucks into the African bush and saw children who hadn't eaten for days. I saw kids fighting over water bottles and bananas. I also saw children laughing with joy as they ran into the ocean wearing tattered swim clothes. I saw teenagers who told me miraculous stories of food multiplying when they were hungry and prayed over their meals. I saw young people rescued from garbage dumps who are now leaders, preparing for college and careers. I learned that a person's success or value isn't determined by how much money or how many resources they have. We are valued and loved by God because of who we are, not what we have. We are His beloved creation, made in His image and likeness.

Think about the way you view success. What is most important to you? What do you want for your children? What do you think makes someone truly rich? Is prosperity found solely in financial gain? How important are things money can't buy, like family, friendships, and love? You might not be able to provide everything materially that a child can dream of, but you can give them what they need the most—love and support. You can love your child right now by doing everything in your power to keep them safe.

Thirty-nine years after my mom left that abortion clinic, I am a mother, a wife, and a minister at my church. I have experienced loving and lasting relationships with friends and family. I graduated from college and spent years doing mission work. I have traveled to parts of Africa, Nepal, Italy, Guatemala, Holland, and all around this nation. I have worked with the elderly and with children, mentored teens, and spent four years aiding women and their families at a pregnancy center. I have done outreaches in poverty-stricken places and was in a meeting at the Oval Office of the White House. I have a beautiful home and I am blessed to live just minutes away from my mother. Andrea is now a grandmother who comes over often to help me with my baby and to spend time together. She is able to be a loving grandmother to my son because she said yes to keeping me. All that I have done in my nearly forty years was possible because my mother choose life over abortion. The words the kind janitor gave her decades ago are the same words I say to you today. *God will give you the strength to have this baby.*

Resources to Find Help

In the places where you struggle to provide, there are resources available to you. Here is some information on pregnancy centers, food, housing, and healthcare options. For other needs, additional resources and information are available at www.allayresources.com.

Pregnancy Resource Centers

Care Net

With more than 1,100 affiliates across North America, chances are there is a Care Net pregnancy center in your community, ready and equipped to serve you.

Free services you can receive at your local center may include:

- Free pregnancy tests
- STD/STI testing and information
- Limited obstetrical ultrasound services
- Parenting programs
- Options information, including both abortion and carrying your baby to term.

Care Net is available to talk Monday through Friday, 10:00 a.m.–6:00 p.m. (EST). You can ask them anything; they are here for you. Call 877-791-5475 or go online to https://resources.care-net.org/find-a-pregnancy-center/.

Heartbeat International

"Heartbeat International is the first network of pro-life pregnancy resource centers in the U.S. and the largest and most expansive in the world. . . . We are a nonprofit, interdenominational Christian association of faith-based pregnancy resource centers, medical clinics, maternity homes, and nonprofit adoption agencies endorsed by Christian leaders nationwide." If you are pregnant and in need of immediate assistance, call their 24/7 helpline at (800) 712-HELP (800-712-4357) or visit https://optionline.org.

Birthright

Birthright is committed to providing confidential, non-judgmental support to any woman who is pregnant or thinks she might be pregnant, no matter her age, race, circumstances, religion, marital status, or financial situation. Along with providing love and support, they help with essentials such as pregnancy testing, medical, housing and counseling referrals, as well as maternity and baby items. Their free and confidential helpline is available 24/7 at (800) 550-4900 or visit https://birthright.org/.

Food

Feeding America

The Feeding America network is the nation's largest domestic hunger-relief organization, working to connect people with food and end hunger. Find your local food bank using Feeding America's helpful food bank locator at https://www.feedingamerica.org/ or http://feedingamerica.org/foodbank-results.aspx. They can also be contacted at https://www.facebook.com/FeedingAmerica/ and by phone at (800) 771-2303.

Supplemental Nutrition Assistance Program (SNAP)

If eligible, the SNAP program will help pay your grocery bill so that you and your child can eat well while you attend school. To be eligible, students must be a single parent who has a child under the age of six years in the home. The applicant may not have over $2,000 in cash or bank account assets. Student loans do not count as assets. For more information, go to https://www.fns.usda.gov/snap/supplemental-nutrition-assistance-program.

Special Supplemental Nutrition Program for Women, Infants, and Children (WIC)

The Special Supplemental Nutrition Program for Women, Infants, and Children (WIC) provides federal grants to states for supplemental foods, health care referrals, and nutrition education for low-income pregnant, breastfeeding, and non-breastfeeding postpartum women, and to infants and children up to age five who are found to be at nutritional risk. For more information, go to https://www.fns.usda.gov/wic/women-infants-and-children. To apply, go to https://www.fns.usda.gov/wic/wic-how-apply. To contact your WIC state agency, go to https://www.fns.usda.gov/wic/toll-free-numbers-wic-state-agencies.

Food Pantries

Food pantries are charitable organizations that distribute food to those who have difficulty providing for themselves. Food pantries are not associated with any government agency or any particular nonprofit organization. Food pantries are located throughout the United States. For help locating a local food pantry near you, go to http://www.foodpantries.org/.

Housing

HUD Rental Assistance

The US Department of Housing and Urban Development (HUD) helps apartment owners offer reduced rents to low-income tenants by subsidizing privately owned housing. Interested tenants can search for an apartment at https://resources.hud.gov/. They should then apply directly at the management office. Qualified applicants can also take advantage in the Housing Choice Voucher Program (Section 8). This allows participants to find their own place to live and then to use the voucher to pay for all or part of the rent. To apply, contact a public housing agency. For more information about HUD rental assistance programs, go to https://www.hud.gov/topics/rental_assistance, contact a housing counseling agency, or call toll-free (800) 569-4287.

Catholic Charities

Catholic Charities is committed to helping people, regardless of their faith, who are struggling with poverty and other complex issues. For more information, go to https://www.catholiccharitiesusa.org/, https://www.facebook.com/catholiccharitiesusa/, or call (703) 549-1390.

DomesticShelters.org

If you are suffering from physical, emotional, psychological, or verbal abuse, Domestic Shelters can help you find a nearby shelter and domestic violence program. This free service provides verified information about shelters across the country. For more information, go to https://www.domesticshelters.org/ or https://www.facebook.com/domesticshelters.

National Maternity Housing Coalition

The mission of the National Maternity Housing Coalition is to inspire excellence among maternity housing providers and articulate a collective voice to advance the culture of life and the gospel of Jesus Christ. For more information, go to https://natlhousingcoalition.org/, https://www.facebook.com/NationalMaternityHousingCoalition, call (800) 712-4357, or email housing@heartbeatinternational.org.

Healthcare

Federally Qualified Health Centers (FQHCs) and Rural Health Centers (RHCs)

There are over 13,500 federally qualified health centers (FQHCs) and rural health centers (RHCs) available in the United States. Both types of centers are required by federal law to provide low-cost health care to medically underserved areas (MUA) of the country, regardless of a client's ability to pay. They accept Medicaid and Medicare insurance plans, and they cannot turn away a client who is unable to pay for services. FQHCs must provide services on a sliding fee scale with varying discounts available (based on patient family size and income in accordance with federal poverty guidelines). And each center is required to provide comprehensive primary and preventative care services. By law, they cannot provide abortion services. To find a health center, go to https://findahealthcenter.hrsa.gov/ or http://getyourcare.org/.

13

But God Intended It for Good: Finding Purpose in Pregnancy from Rape

—Paula Ilari—

My story begins with trauma, but doesn't end there. It is a story of God's redemption, love, and mercy after a rape that temporarily left me unable to see that my life still had purpose.

That Saturday in January began like any other. I spent the afternoon catching up with a friend from college. We met at a Mexican restaurant and had an early meal, chatting over queso and guacamole. After we left the restaurant, we stopped to get matching tattoos. A portion of my arm had to be covered in a bandage and a top layer of plastic wrap to keep the wound clean. That would not be the most painful wound inflicted on me that night. But much like the tattoo, my deeper scars would eventually heal.

The Assault

Throughout that afternoon, I had been texting back and forth with a guy another friend thought would be a good match for me. I did not know him well, but my friend had vouched for him, having told me about how great of a person he was, someone she had first met in high school. I trusted her judgment. I shouldn't have.

When he texted me to ask if I wanted to come over and watch television late that Saturday evening, it seemed harmless enough.

I remember that the apartment was cold. We sat on the couch. He flipped on the TV, landing on a show I had never seen before and that didn't catch my interest. Then he tossed the remote aside, kissed me, and began touching me. Instantly uncomfortable, I pulled away. This was a first date. I wasn't looking for anything serious, and certainly no part of me desired to become intimate with someone I was just meeting for the first time. I'd made romantic mistakes in the past and had dealt with the emotional consequences of those poor choices. I had decided months before that I'd do things differently when I began dating again.

His advances continued. As he touched me again, I responded by telling him that I wasn't ready and pulled away once more. He continued to get more and more handsy, prompting me to stand up to leave. I was annoyed and just wanted to go home. But as I made my way to the front door, the guy's roommate came out of a bedroom and blocked the way to the door. My "date" said coldly, "I don't think you're going anywhere right now."

Sometimes I can still feel the squeeze of his arm pressed against me, his roughness, his smell. I thought I was going to die. Part of me even thought it would be easier if I had, because what happened next was not a reality anyone would want to live with. The two of them raped and sodomized me. I don't remember the exact moment, but at some point, that part of me deep inside that made me who I was vanished. When they finished with me, they told me I could go. My "date" followed me outside and thanked me "for a great time." I wrapped my coat around me as tightly as I could and stumbled to my car. The cheerful, twenty-four-year-old woman who walked into that apartment was not the same person who walked out.

The Aftermath

The door locks clicked, and I put the car in reverse to back out of the parking spot. I don't have any recollection of the first half of my drive home. Suddenly, I did not want to be alone. I was on the interstate, and I fumbled around with my phone for a minute. After trying to reach two of the people closest to me with no luck, I realized it was by now the middle of the night and I gave up trying to make calls.

When I got home, I was fixated on getting clean. Not just bathing, but scrubbing. My body was sore, and I felt as though my entire being was covered in a kind of filth that wouldn't come off, no matter how much hot water and soap I added to the equation. Eventually, I crumbled to the shower floor, my behind hitting the bottom of the tub around the same time as my tears. It seemed as though I drifted back and forth between being completely numb and being overwhelmed with emotion. When a bottle of body wash slipped off the side of the tub and fell in beside me, I threw it against the shower wall. In that moment, it felt cruel for God to allow me to live.

"You should have let them kill me! Why didn't they just kill me?!" I raged. There was no answer.

A blur of hours passed, and I still didn't want to be alone. After making the decision to go to that man's apartment, I couldn't trust myself to think straight. It was now Sunday, and I just wanted to be at church. So many of my good friends would be there, including "Dee," an especially close friend though several years older, a woman on staff at the church. It was she I wanted to talk with. I felt completely safe around her and I could tell her what had happened. I wanted her to fix things, as if anyone could ever "fix" the aftermath of rape.

I don't remember getting ready or driving to church, but when I think of it, I can still feel the way the cold January air hit my cheeks as I walked toward the red door that marked the church's entrance. I found Dee, and we talked briefly before the service. The conversation is a bit of a blur, but she asked some questions and listened. Then she suggested we get coffee after church if I felt like I could stay and make it through the service. The music comforted me, though I have no recollection whatsoever of the sermon.

On the way to the coffee shop, we stopped at a drug store, where Dee told me we needed to take care of something important. She led me to the family planning aisle and handed me a box of Plan B, otherwise known as the morning-after pill. I had described myself previously as "personally pro-life and politically pro-choice." I knew having an abortion wasn't something I ever wanted to do, but around that time, I was somewhere in the middle of shifting closer to a pro-life stance—no longer pro-choice, but not yet ready to fully embrace the pro-life label. I wasn't sure how to tell Dee that I didn't want to take that pill.

I knew how it worked. The morning-after pill could either prevent ovulation or keep a fertilized embryo from implanting into the uterus if ovulation had taken place. But the emotional state I was in already had me feeling overwhelmed. I didn't feel up to a discussion about abortifacient drugs, so I said I wanted to go on to the coffee shop.

The thought of being alone still made me feel vulnerable. Despite the detour to Walgreens, I needed to be with a good friend, someone I trusted more than I could trust myself just then.

Caramel macchiato for me. Dee ordered a bagel with lox. We sat down at a table slightly more secluded than the rest, and when we got settled, she encouraged me to take the Plan B. I pushed it off again: "Maybe in a little while."

"You really need this. It's important to take it soon."

As we talked, Dee continued to tell me how imperative it was that I take the pill right then. I mentioned not being sure I would, and that just made her more determined to convince me. When we left the coffee shop and I still hadn't taken it, she spent the next couple of days texting me about it, then calling. If I didn't answer she'd leave voice mails all with the same message: her worry that I hadn't taken the Plan B option, and that the three-day window was soon to close.

And I did briefly consider it. My mind was so cluttered. I felt like it was more responsible to try to ignore my feelings so that I could make a logical decision, but I couldn't rid myself of the knowledge that it was wrong. The decision was made. I wouldn't take that pill.

I didn't feel like explaining myself, so I avoided the continued texts and calls from Dee, which came with increasing frequency for a few days. Once the 72 hours to take the drug had passed, the voicemails went from pressuring me to take it to inquiring whether I had.

I spiraled further into depression. I couldn't see myself as worthy or valuable. I felt nasty—like I was all used up. My daily existence seemed more like a funeral than a life. I mourned the loss of who I was, and my grief was slowly drowning me. I didn't know why I was allowed to live, but death seemed like the only escape from the reality of what had happened to me. I did the only thing I could do—I just held on.[1]

The Smile

Two weeks went by. I woke up that Saturday morning and just felt strange—the kind of strange that sent me to Walgreens, where I exchanged the unopened box of Plan B for a box of digital pregnancy tests.

It seems like such an out-of-body experience: the drive to the store, the transaction, the chitchat with the cashier, the drive home, the walk into the bathroom, the instructions on the box, taking the test. But truthfully, I had not felt fully present since the rape. My physical body was the site of a disaster, like an island devastated by a tsunami. Sometimes the losses we experience make it impossible to go back to what we were. Perhaps our minds protect us by erecting a barrier to raw emotions. I felt that way that day.

There I sat in the bathroom, completely destroyed inside, holding a pregnancy test.

And then the trajectory shifted. The positive result appeared, and I smiled. It was the first time since being raped that I had felt any semblance of joy. In that moment, everything changed. I finally understood why I was alive. God hadn't orchestrated my pain, but He had allowed me to live through that night so that He could use my life for a purpose. I knew I had to keep living, and now I was excited to do so, because somebody else was depending on me. My baby saved me the very moment I learned of his existence. I needed to feel needed, valuable, like my life still had purpose. God filled each need with His creation.

The Pressure

The next morning, I went to church. I had not stopped smiling yet. When I ran into Dee, she asked why I hadn't responded to her many calls and texts and wanted to be assured I had taken the medication.

"No," I said, still smiling. "And I'm pregnant."

She seemed shocked and confused about how I could possibly be happy about this news. "What are you going to do?" she asked, but in a way that made it clear she expected to hear me respond with the name of an abortion clinic and an appointment time.

I simply said, "I'm choosing joy."

Throughout my pregnancy, I gave that response to countless others when they would ask the same question in the same manner. From the very beginning, it was a struggle. Dee actually stopped speaking to me because I wouldn't consider abortion. A few others followed her lead, but for the most part, people took up the challenge of pressuring me into having the abortion I had repeatedly said I did not want. It was intense and overwhelming. I received continuous phone calls, voicemails, texts, and social media messages. It became clear to me that so-called choice was nothing more than a myth, for those who would describe themselves as being pro-choice completely refused to accept the firm decision I had made.

My pregnancy was not an easy one physically, either. Due to an infection stemming from the rape, I bled heavily for most of the first two trimesters (from about 4.5 weeks until 19 weeks and 6 days). It took months to discover the infection and multiple rounds of antibiotics to clear it up. I was terrified. The bleeding would become so heavy that the on-call doctor repeatedly directed me to the emergency room to be evaluated for a potential miscarriage. Other times, I was seen in my obstetrician's office during regular hours. I lived in fear all day, every day, that I might lose the one person I loved most.

All the while, the "friends" who would still speak to me would do so only to tell me what a huge mistake I was making by not having an abortion. They would say things like:

"That 'thing' is evil."

"It's the spawn of Satan."

"Abort it."

"You know he'll have his dad's DNA, right? You really want to bring another rapist into the world?"

"Get rid of the devil baby."

Those were the milder comments, and they cut through me like a knife.

Most people would find it hard to imagine: all these people who identified as Christian demanding that I have my baby killed, while I was begging God to just let him live. Some days the pain was so intense that I couldn't find the words to speak, and I would sit in the bathroom and pray, prayers consisting mainly of tears. That experience was, no doubt, more traumatic than the gang rape itself.

One of the things that helped me persevere was that I knew something my "friends" did not. To the people at church, I was what they called an "angel." I was the one who donated huge amounts of my time for service projects and gladly babysat for free. I was the one greatly appreciated by everyone in the church—staff and laypeople alike—for all I did.

But what they didn't know was that I carried a shameful secret: *I, too, had been conceived in rape when my birth mother was assaulted at knifepoint in 1991*. People were so sure that no one conceived in rape could ever grow up to be a decent human being—how surprised they would be if they knew that someone they so adored had had such a beginning to her existence.

Being able to see the inconsistencies between their statements and my own lived experiences made it easier for me to keep going, but the ongoing harassment was nearly unbearable. I was calling my son by the name I had chosen for him—Caleb—for weeks while still being met with offers to arrange a late-term abortion procedure. "It's not too late to fix this." I lost count of how many people said that to me. But it never hurt as much as it did the night a group of women invited me to a "baby shower," only for me to arrive and discover it was an intervention designed as a last-ditch effort to convince me to have a late-term abortion.

Their idea of support involved pushing me into a violent procedure that would have taken the life of my baby, whose existence was the only reason I had for continuing to live. The only real and consistent support I encountered came from my pro-life obstetrician and her all-female staff. Simply allowing me to have a safe space to chat excitedly about my son's life, offering me a smile, and being genuinely kind meant more than any of them could have imagined.

When someone asked me to speak with a woman who could offer resources to single moms, I agreed. I knew I could benefit from some assistance, so I scheduled the meeting. When the woman arrived at the restaurant, we sat down to talk. A couple of minutes into the conversation, I realized this woman would indeed offer me help, but only if I agreed to place my son for adoption. I believe adoption is a wonderful option for many women, but it was not the right choice for me. It became increasingly clear that this woman was not at all interested in my well-being. I ended the meeting and left.

The Arrival

It was at this point that I shut down a little more. I kept to myself as much as possible and didn't talk to very many people. Realizing I would be alone when I delivered my baby, I hired a doula. None of my friends offered to be present with me during labor, and nobody else showed up at the hospital to offer to support me the day my baby arrived. Everyone in that delivery room was paid to be there, a reality I'm still saddened to remember.

During my labor—literally mid-contraction—two women walked into my room uninvited. They introduced themselves as social workers from the hospital and asked if I'd let the family know yet that I was in labor.

"Huh? What family?" I asked.

"The adoptive family," the older one replied.

I was so confused. "What? He's mine. I'm not placing him for adoption."

"Oh, honey," she said, "in these situations, you're just better off without the reminder."

The details of what I said in response aren't important. They also do not showcase my love for Jesus, if I'm being honest. Let's just say these social workers were promptly told to leave before I physically removed them from the room. I'd had enough of people browbeating me about *my* situation, *my* life, and *my* baby. I'd had enough of them telling me what I *had* to do and what I *needed* when they knew absolutely nothing about either.

The hands on the clock hanging high up on the wall continued to move forward, as did my labor. Before long, I was pushing. With the massive load of adrenaline I had built up over the prior nine months, it didn't seem to take much exertion to birth my beautiful 7-pound, 10-ounce baby boy. He came out crying and settled down when they placed him on my chest.

I finally had the privilege of holding all the happiness in the world in my own two arms. Names have always been of interest to me, and I was intentional about the name I had chosen for Caleb. His first and two middle names together mean "wholehearted, honorable gift of God." It was important that his name carry a message of how I had always felt about him, just in case he ever doubted my love because of the foolishness of others.

And foolish they were. I assumed people would change their minds when they met the baby, and while some previously outspoken individuals did get very quiet, many remained adamant that I had made a grave mistake in both carrying and parenting my son. These women never missed an opportunity to make me feel small or to remind me that they saw us as being drastically different from other single-parent families. As I walked through the church sanctuary with my newborn in his carrier and large bags looming under my eyes one Sunday, one of the women who had participated in the fake baby shower asked how I was doing.

"Just a little tired," I replied. Newborns don't sleep much, and I clearly was not the first, the millionth, or the last to have the experience of sleep deprivation after giving birth.

"Well," she said, "I don't feel sorry for you. You knew exactly what this would be like when you decided to keep that thing!" As soon as the words left her mouth, she walked away.

The lack of support was palpable. There were no meal deliveries, no offers of help—nothing. A large group of people knew I was entering motherhood completely alone, and they intentionally left me that way.

Redemption

Fortunately, we have a loving God who never abandons us. He spared my life the night I was gang-raped and saved me again with the gift of my son. He was with me for the duration of my pregnancy, and He held me together after Caleb's birth. Since then, He has called me into ministry work and offered me opportunities to share our story and help others, both of which have helped me heal in ways I couldn't have imagined over the last several years.

It has been over five years since I was gang-raped, and my life is full and blessed. I met and married my husband in 2020. He is a wonderful man who saw Caleb and me as a package deal—the two missing pieces in his life. His parents were excited to become instant grandparents, and their entire extended family quickly embraced us. We had our second little boy in 2021, and Caleb is the best, most adoring big brother. We now attend a loving, life-affirming church, where my family and my ministry are both supported by those in the congregation. In the weeks and months after the rape, if someone had asked me whether or not I would ever live this kind of life, I would have thought they were crazy. But God is still in the miracle business.

I like to keep pictures on my desk. The most prominent is a family shot of Caleb being held by my husband, who is standing next to me, and our baby boy in my arms. That photo showcases the beautiful ways God works all things for our good (Rom. 8:28). There are other photographs: pictures of Caleb playing, ultrasound pictures of his baby brother, and a photo of me with a student from the school where I used to work. Each brings a smile to my face, and none of those moments would have happened without God's provision.

I also keep a picture of another little girl, whose teenage mother I had the privilege of helping after she became pregnant from rape. She reminds me about why I can't hide the truth of our story, why I must speak loudly and without hesitation. Other lives, like hers, hang in the balance, and I have a duty to share with other moms what God has done in my life and will do in theirs. My own healing has had a ripple effect in the lives of others—the families I have come to know and journey with as they have navigated their own situations involving rape conception.

The story of our family began with trauma, but, as I mentioned earlier, it doesn't end there. If I had given in to the pressure to choose abortion, I—and any future family—would only have endured even more trauma. My favorite Bible verse is Genesis 50:20 (NIV), which reads, "You intended to harm me, but God intended it for good to accomplish what is now being done, the saving of many lives."

My life was the first life saved. Caleb's was the second. It isn't possible for me to know how many more have been saved since. That's the real story of our family—one highlighting the saving grace of God and the ability of His love to take our deepest pain and give it immense purpose.

Encouragement

If you, reader, are pregnant after being raped, I first want to say that I am so sorry you were violated in this way. I am thankful you are safe, and I hope you connect with my ministry, Hope After Rape Conception,[2] so that we can help connect you with support and you can begin to heal.

Though there are far too many uneducated people who don't understand why, you are not crazy for loving your baby. In a major study on the subject, Amy Sobie and David Reardon found that 73 percent of women pregnant from rape choose life. Of those 73 percent, 64 percent choose to parent, and 36 percent make an adoption plan. Of the women who had abortions, 98 percent expressed regret.[3] The numbers don't lie. It is natural and normal for women to love our babies, no matter how they were conceived. It goes completely against our natural instincts to pursue abortion. We would never be allowed or pressured to kill our rapists. Why should our children be penalized for a crime they never committed?

Whatever stage of grief you are walking through right now, please know that there are women, like me, who have already walked this road, just waiting to journey with you. The dark days do not last forever. Better days are coming, and amazing days will follow them. You and your baby have untold joy ahead. God is already working to transform your pain into purpose.

Even though your story begins with trauma, it is not over. You have arrived at a beautiful, new beginning.

14

Fearfully and Wonderfully Made: Reimagining Pregnancy When the Baby Has Disabilities

—Carlynn Fabarez—

After ten years of marriage, three and a half years of infertility, three surgeries, and countless medical treatments, my husband, Mike, and I welcomed our first baby—a boy we named Matthew. Less than two years later I gave birth to his brother, John. Another year later, after we had prayed to add one more child to fill the chairs around our kitchen table, we soon learned my infertility had returned. The next couple of years were a familiar roller coaster, which included months of disappointment, another surgery, and a full round of medical treatments.

On the very day my husband and I had decided to be content with our family of four, we discovered I was pregnant. It was a day of rejoicing, but the joy gave way to sickness—a kind of trying sickness that I had not known with my other two pregnancies. In the fourth month I went in for a routine ultrasound to learn if the baby would be a little brother or a little sister for Matthew and John. Even with the change from the previous asymptomatic pregnancies to the rocky journey I had been experiencing, we had zero expectation of the news that would soon completely rock our world.

Mike took time off from work to join me for what we fully anticipated would be a joyful gender reveal appointment. Midway through the grainy hunt for our child's telling anatomy, our ultrasound technician quickly excused herself. Her crestfallen face was clear. Something was wrong. Seriously wrong. After what seemed like an excruciatingly long wait, the doctor walked in, picked up the wand, pointed to the screen, and began to explain the blurry image. As he directed the field of focus to our child's spinal cord, which to us looked like a tiny string of pearls, he moved up the spine, stopped and said, "That! That dark spot right there. That should not be there." Then the news got worse.

The doctor slowly moved the screen's view up our baby's back, he reached the head and said, "And all of that. It shouldn't be dark like that." He removed the wand from my belly, and in a sobering tone explained that our baby had a serious neural tube defect, which had not allowed the spinal cord to "zip up" properly—commonly known as spina bifida. Worse, he said the most serious problem was with the brain, or in this case, the seeming lack thereof. That was the first time I heard the word *anencephaly*—a condition wherein the baby's brain is not developed, resulting in blindness, deafness, and stillbirth in three out of four cases. We were devastated.

"By the way," we were told in the midst of it all, "it's a girl." Then he quickly went on to tell us that it was time to talk to a geneticist and to schedule an abortion. In a matter of fifteen minutes our world was turned upside down.

The Push for an Abortion

The doctor was adamant. There was only one choice here: "The fetus needs to be aborted," he plainly and matter-of-factly stated. It was amazing to us how quickly the appointment went from an environment where a friendly tech was eagerly wanting to share in our joy and excitement about the gender discovery of our new baby, to a swift and hurried push to schedule the disposal of this hopelessly damaged "growth" in my body. The change in tone was jarring.

By this time in our lives Mike had been pastoring a church in our southern California town for years. He had walked many families through their trials, losses, challenges, and pains. And of course, we had both had plenty of opportunities to help counsel, guide, and carry the burdens of those walking through all kinds of diseases, disabilities, and losses in the wake of death.

The doctor's emphatic words were like fingers on a chalkboard, yet we instinctively engaged our theological commitments with a resolve that abortion would not be an option. We spoke up immediately and told him that we had no interest in hearing any more about it. The doctor firmly stated that while he assumed we were "philosophically opposed" to the procedure, it really was in the best interest of everyone involved. Either way, he told us, we needed to immediately schedule an appointment with a geneticist to answer a series of questions about our family tree, our parents' health, and to acquire more information about the path and options that lay before us.

The meeting with the geneticist was more of the same. We encountered firm, professional counsel to see the virtue of ending the pregnancy. But to us it wasn't just a pregnancy. It, of course, was our child. Our daughter. A daughter my husband and I had immaturely named while dating in high school. The timing for naming our daughter may have been silly, but twenty years later the choice still seemed like the right one—her name would be *Stephanie.*

Stephanie's life was in peril. That's how we understood the news, which of course was exactly what we had been told. The professionals told us that she likely wouldn't live to full term. The doctors told us that even if she were to survive for hours or days outside the womb, it would never be a life worth living. Either way, our hearts went out to our Stephanie, and even if my body would be the only home she would ever know, we were determined that it would be free from the intrusion of the abortionist's tools.

When the news got out about Stephanie's prognosis, we received much support and encouragement to strengthen and prepare us for the dark days ahead. But to our surprise, the loud voices of our shifting culture on the topic of abortion had an impact on even those in our close circles. The concern about a life not worth living, and the call to minimize the pain in this world, and the fears of costs and compounded suffering led some to join the medical voices—whispering that it really would "be best" if we would just end our daughter's life.

When pious-sounding churchgoers told us that our daughter's life was "a mistake," and that she was "clearly broken," and we should accept our parental duty to "fix the problem," we realized that "choosing life" in modern America was a more unpopular decision than we had anticipated—even within the Christian subculture.

Revisiting a Commitment to Preborn Life

Now more than ever we would all do well to reaffirm the reasons for choosing life for the preborn regardless of the prenatal diagnoses. It was good for me, in our darkest days, to return to the reasons that a trip to the doctor's office cannot change the reality of human life and its sanctity. And I pray that considering the following ten reasons to choose life will also strengthen your resolve when fear and uncertainty assault your heart.

1. The Diagnosis May Be Wrong

Even in our day of advanced medical technology and expensive diagnostic testing, the diagnoses of severe birth defects are often inaccurate. Consider these facts about screening results that often trigger the shift of a mom's valuation of her preborn child from a precious life to a mass of defective tissue. Current medical professionals admit that:

> About 50 women out of every 1,000 [or 3–5%] will have a result on the quad screen (or AFP blood test) that indicates an increased risk of a birth defect, but only one to two (or 2–4%) of those women will actually have a baby with an open neural tube defect. And about 40 women out of 1,000 [or 4%] will have a result indicating an increased risk of Down syndrome, but only one to two [3–5%] of these women will have a baby with Down syndrome.[1]

While Stephanie's initial diagnosis was almost two decades ago, the hopeless conclusion, and the bleak prognosis of "possibly surviving only for a few hours outside the womb," were in fact wildly pessimistic and clearly inaccurate. Our daughter, who has battled spina bifida her whole life, is now battling her first set of college assignments—just like all of her fellow freshmen.

2. Human Worth Is Never Determined by Abilities

Even when the diagnosis is accurate or the reality is worse than the doctors expected, it is important to return to the basic affirmation that your life, my life, and your preborn child's life is not holy, special, or worth living simply because we are capable of doing this task or accomplishing certain goals. Recall the celebration of human life made in God's image—regardless of intelligence, competencies, or abilities.

> For you formed my inward parts;
>   you knitted me together in my mother's womb.
> I praise you, for I am fearfully and wonderfully made.
> Wonderful are your works;
>   my soul knows it very well.
>   My frame was not hidden from you,
>   when I was being made in secret,
>   intricately woven in the depths of the earth.
> Your eyes saw my unformed substance;
> in your book were written, every one of them,
>   the days that were formed for me,
>   when as yet there was none of them. (Ps. 139:13–16)

God goes even further, taking upon Himself the ultimate responsibility for the capacities and limitations of all human life. He counts imperfect lives as precious and worthy of His redemptive love when He asks Moses, "Who has made man's mouth? Who makes him mute, or deaf, or seeing, or blind? Is it not I, the LORD?" (Ex. 4:11). Affirming the sovereignty of God even in the most severely curtailing circumstances is a good start in knowing life does not become worthy of living when it crosses a threshold of performance or capacity.

Actually, to fail to think in these terms (as so many inadvertently do) is to agree with the reasoning of leaders in Nazi Germany, who forged a set of values to determine when a life was worthy of being granted life.[2] The atrocities of herding people into gas chambers or systematically executing the sick, disabled, and all those deemed "useless" is not materially different from the prevailing views of aborting our "broken" preborn children.

In our early dark days, my husband would seek to point out the logic of our critics who were pushing for the abortion of Stephanie with the line, "We will try her out for a couple of years and if she is not able to do everything we had hoped, we will just put her down then." It may have seemed defensive, but it clearly made the point: the worth of human life is never determined by abilities.

3. *Minimizing My Baby's Suffering Is Not Grounds for Killing Her*

The words "do no harm," found in the traditional recitation of the Hippocratic Oath and still pledged by many entering the medical profession today, could serve as what we should hope is an unnecessary reminder of a mother's commitment to her child. Like the ER doctor who never knows what may be wheeled in through the doors at 2:00 a.m., the goal is to deal with whatever "brokenness" lies before her, and then diligently proceed to do what can be done to fix it.

A mother's concession to the new values of so many of today's medical professionals to see the "brokenness" of defects or disabilities, and then proceed to eliminate the suffering by killing the patient, should be seen for what it is—moral insanity. No parent asks for a child who has greater pains, discomforts, or limitations than other children, but like the moral ER doctor who knows his task is to help and not to harm, we are all called to roll up our sleeves and be agents of assistance to those who are suffering.

Broad and regular mercy killing of children and adults in our society may be closer than we want to believe, in part because the same logic has been legally taking place in the womb for decades. Our submission to the command to "not murder" (Ex. 20:13) cannot be set aside because we decide someone's life is, or will be, in too much pain. Our preborn children need our help, not our efforts to dismember and dispose of them.

4. Abortion Cannot Be the Means to Minimize My Suffering

In the middle of a sleepless night, as a mom begins to process the terrifying diagnosis of a critically ill preborn child, the ultimate internal battle is viciously waged. Questions swirl through a mom's head: What will this do to my family? Can I really take care of this child? What stress will this put on my marriage? How will I be able to endure all of the challenges? What will this cost? Can we afford it? Can I live with the pain and disappointment of having a critically ill child?

And of course, most in our society have a quick and convenient solution: abortion! There's your quick fix. All the looming threats can be terminated, along with the life of this "broken mass of tissue." It can be over. All that anticipation of struggle and personal suffering can be gone with the scheduling of a single appointment at the clinic.

These private temptations must be honestly faced. And the

"solution" of abortion must be truthfully evaluated. The pain and grief will not be eliminated, they will only be shifted. And in light of the facts, the logic, the theology, and the truth of what this kind of mercy killing actually is, the pain is markedly worse. The decision to end the life of your child with disabilities may be internally rationalized, but as Scripture so clearly states, we should "not be deceived: God is not mocked, for whatever one sows, that will he also reap" (Gal. 6:7). Randy Alcorn shows how, even when repentance and divine forgiveness for murder is sought, the psychological consequences often remain: "One study showed that of forty-eight women who terminated their pregnancies for genetic reasons, 77 percent demonstrated acute grief reactions, and 45 percent continued in this grief six months after the abortion. Another study showed a higher rate of depression for genetic abortion than for other kinds, and demonstrated postabortion family disharmony and flashbacks."[3]

Even when genetic factors end a child's life within hours or days of birth, the nobility of seeking to help and not harm guards your conscience. Family and friends can walk you through the grief. You will not regret holding your baby, naming your baby, and if need be, giving your baby a respectful and dignified goodbye. Each of these steps can be incredibly helpful in the grieving process. Even if your body is the only home your child will ever know, you can experience the peace amid the pain, that your strength and decisions did all that could be done to protect and assist your baby.

5. Abortion Is Not Fixing God's Mistakes

Even in reading the above statement, I trust you can see the presumption of such logic. Not only does such a suggestion clearly contradict God's words to Moses—namely by suggesting that those born with disabilities are "God's mistakes" (recall Ex. 4:11)—but it also implies that the disposal of a preborn child can help God along to make things right.

Again, we must underscore the sovereignty of God. While God will one day make all things right, the wrong in this world is not outside of God's strategic management. If we are to believe anything in the Bible, we must believe that disappointing setbacks and painful detours are all part of God's carefully crafted plan for our lives.

When Abraham and Sarah were promised and purposed by God to be the ancestors of a great nation with countless citizens, they were an aging, infertile couple. And when God gave them this promise, one would think that in the next verse they'd be preparing for the arrival of their firstborn. But God didn't make them wait nine months, or even nine years. God provided them with a personally crafted detour that took them down the road twenty-five long and painful years.

Why? God had a plan. And all the attempts to "help God along" and "fix the problem" of childlessness were seen as folly. Coveting, jealousy, anger, betrayal, and heartache were experienced because they rushed to fix a perceived problem in God's plan.

Instead of intervening with the immoral rush to end a child's life that we have concluded is "God's mistake" or "God's failure," let us stand with Job in his initial response to the tragic setbacks in his life. Let us say with him, "shall we receive good from God, and shall we not receive evil?" (Job 2:10). Few people hate the evil of infertility or birth defects more than I do, but I hope that we can worshipfully receive the lot from God that He has personally chosen for each of us.

6. God Is Working All Things Together for Good

The maturity all Christians seek is quickly tested by our ability to wholeheartedly concur with the remarkable truth that for those who love our sovereign God, "all things work together for good, for those who are called according to his purpose" (Rom. 8:28). We must know that the "all" includes the painful prenatal diagnosis of a child with disabilities.

Agreement with this divine declaration is a realization that God has chosen this path for us and our family. While surprising to us, it is not a surprise to the Lord. It was wisely chosen for the working of good. This will be a test of our faith, as we are told in 1 Peter 1:6–7. And while admittedly grievous (v. 6), it is designed to "result in praise and glory and honor," if not in the short run, then without question "at the revelation of Jesus Christ" (v. 7).

When the man with the congenital birth defect that had left him blind his entire life was encountered by the disciples in John 9, the natural question for those believing in the God who controls every molecule of the universe was posed. They asked, "Why?" They mused about why God would assign such an apparent evil thing to this family. They said, "Who sinned, this man or his parents, that he was born blind?" (v. 2). Jesus said it was neither, but so "that the works of God might be displayed in him" (v. 3).

God had a specific and superior reason for taking this man and his parents through all the years of pain, struggle, and disadvantage. God had designed this evil to be used for the good of Christ's convincing and authenticating encounter with the whole family, which was recorded and has been used in the lives of millions of people through the centuries. This man's disability led him and many others to the forgiveness of sins and the assurance of eternal life.

While it would be silly even to try to compare the far-reaching effects of that family's trials to our own, I can certainly testify that the good which God has and is still producing through the disability of our beloved Stephanie is noteworthy in my little corner of the world. My daughter's birth defects have been the cause for much good fruit in this world, as have the lives of so many others with disabilities we have come to know over the years. God certainly works all things together for good.

7. People with Disabilities Contribute Much Good in This World

The grace of life is extended by God to the smart and the simple, the weak and the strong, the beautiful and the plain. And with that grace comes good, which God is always producing in and through the almost endless variety He has ordained in His creation. Those who so quickly assume that a disabling prognosis would be nothing more than a drain on society and therefore not worthy of life ought to work to recall how God has greatly benefited our world through the ages by those who, in our day, would likely be discarded had their limitations been discovered prenatally.

Helen Keller was blind. Edison was hard of hearing (he lost most of his hearing around the age of twelve). Physical limitations haven't deprived us of Perlman's violin, Franklin Roosevelt's presidency, Beethoven's concertos, or Einstein's contributions to discovering the laws of God's creation. The good health and physical prowess of Ted Bundy, Osama bin Laden, Timothy McVeigh, or Adolf Hitler certainly didn't provide us the good we pray for God to produce through our children.

A weekend of reflective conversation with the experienced parents of a mentally challenged child or Down syndrome teen will undoubtedly change your assumptions that what God wants to produce in this world only comes from towering intellects or specimens of physical fitness. God is offering good, grace, and true beauty through a variety of lives, which our uninformed world would encourage us to throw away.

8. Children with Disabilities Experience the Joy of Life

If a mom experiencing a healthy pregnancy and looking forward to a "perfect" child were to stop and consider that her child would in short order experience the discomfort of wet diapers, the excruciating pain of teething, the fear of the first day of school, the ordeal of having a broken bone set, the heartbreak of teenage romance, the frustration of losing a job, the chronic irritation of allergies, the anguish of marital problems, the torment of being sued, the grief of being widowed, then, if her logic about aborting the "imperfect" were to be applied, one could argue that perhaps the future suffering of her "perfect" child should also be mercifully exterminated before all the pain commences.

But of course, no one thinks like that. We focus on the grace of life. We look with anticipation to the joys of life. We imagine and foresee the happy moments that we all know will come amid and between the pain and suffering. It is not different for a child with disabilities. Yes, there is plenty of discomfort, there are surgeries, and there is a lot that hurts. But I can attest that between these challenges there will be good, peace, laughter, and lots of joy. Of course our focus has to be submissive to the call to decide to "rejoice and be glad" in this "day that the LORD has made" (Ps. 118:24); like Job, to decide that were it the worst case scenario, "I will hope in him" (Job 13:15); and purposefully to remember that "The steadfast love of the LORD never ceases; his mercies never come to an end; they are new every morning" because of the greatness of his faithfulness (Lam. 3:22–23). Grace is there. Our job is to decide to recall it, to focus on it, and to celebrate it.

9. Every Disability for the Christian Is Only Temporary

God has told us through the embattled and diseased life of the apostle Paul that all that is wrong in the Christian's life can be summarized under the heading "light and momentary" afflictions (2 Cor. 4:17). Paul believed it, and so should we. Even the most severe and painful experiences are labeled "transient" (v. 18). A child with a serious disability may not seem light, momentary, or transient. But God has said that all "the sufferings of this present time are not worth comparing with the glory that is to be revealed to us" (Rom. 8:18).

It may seem overwhelming and may feel all-consuming, but the pains, problems, and difficulties associated with caring for a child with disabilities are bound to this fleeting and temporary life. Our opportunity to glorify God and accentuate the good He is doing through our trials is the assignment we all have as we make each day count for eternity—which of course highlights the need for everyone, healthy and unhealthy, to heed the call of the gospel to trust in Christ and secure their place in His coming kingdom.

The ultimate joy I continue to celebrate in my daughter's life has not been overcoming her health challenges, or having good news about the outcome of her surgeries, or seeing her mainstreamed in her schools. Instead, it is without question the trust she has placed in Christ as her Savior and Lord. Her disabilities are temporary, but her salvation will be celebrated for eternity.

10. Revel in Your Service to Persons with Disabilities

Discarding the disabled should be unthinkable. Serving them, if that is what God is calling you to, can be your fulfilling joy. When you are given the prenatal prognosis of a critically ill child, you are entering into a job that Jesus freely chose to step into Himself. He made service to the sick, the infirmed, and the diseased a large focus of His earthly work.

Jesus sought out the ill, not only to demonstrate the miraculous authentication of His deity, but also to model for us the way His generous and caring people should live. While we cannot with a word make the lame walk, we can, as Jesus said, serve them. Consider the words of Christ concerning caring for the sick and disabled:

> He said also to the man who had invited him, "When you give a dinner or a banquet, do not invite your friends or your brothers or your relatives or rich neighbors, lest they also invite you in return and you be repaid. But when you give a feast, invite the poor, the crippled, the lame, the blind, and you will be blessed, because they cannot repay you. For you will be repaid at the resurrection of the just." (Luke 14:12–14)

Jesus has called us to not worry about the cost or the fairness or the sacrifice. He reveals in this directive that caring for those who are unable to repay is the sort of expression of love that He himself came to demonstrate.

Even if you are not reading this because you have received a painful diagnosis in your family, follow the prompt of Christ to do what you can to give, serve, and expend yourself for those who are disabled. Our service as Christians is the best kind the world can receive, because our acts of kindness are coupled with the words of life. Our gospel witness to the physically and mentally disadvantaged brings the hope of eternal life.

Strength for the Task

Choosing life when it is especially costly is a responsibility for which God is always faithful to provide. He is the Giver of strength and endurance. The consequences of choosing life will not only provide you with a clear conscience, but with a God who has promised to walk with you through the daily challenges. He has provided His church, and He provides Himself.

Raising a child with disabilities is difficult, but the God who upholds the world can without a doubt uphold you, your family members, and your precious child. He can vanquish fear, calm hearts, and equip you for the task. As you pray, remember the One you address. As you stand with Him for life, recall His infinite power that is able to sustain you. Remember the timeless words He left us through the prophet Isaiah:

> Have you not known? Have you not heard?
> The LORD is the everlasting God,
> the Creator of the ends of the earth.
> He does not faint or grow weary;
> his understanding is unsearchable.
> He gives power to the faint,
> and to him who has no might he increases strength.
> Even youths shall faint and be weary,
> and young men shall fall exhausted;
> but they who wait for the LORD shall renew their strength;
> they shall mount up with wings like eagles;
> they shall run and not be weary;
> they shall walk and not faint. (Isa. 40:28–31)

15

Are Abortions Ever Medically Necessary? A Life-Affirming Approach to Complex Pregnancies

—Kendra Kolb—

It was another typical evening for me in January of 2019, as I prepared a quick dinner for my two small children before my husband came home from work. I had just arrived home after a busy day in the neonatal intensive care unit where I work as a neonatologist, or physician who has been subspecialty trained to care for medically fragile and complex newborns, many of whom are born extremely prematurely, even as early as 22 weeks gestational age. The day had been long, as most of them are, and also emotionally, mentally, and physically demanding, a natural consequence of bearing the weight of responsibility for the well-being of tiny babies, many of whom weigh just over a pound, live in heated incubators, and breathe with the help of ventilators. I became a neonatologist out of my passion for and fascination with these tiny human beings, who never fail to inspire me with their strength and ability to survive outside the womb in spite of their tiny size.

That particular evening, I was on the phone with my mother who, aside from my husband, is my biggest supporter and has encouraged me through the most grueling and challenging times of medical school, residency, and fellowship training. We regularly talk on the phone, particularly after a long day of work. On this night we were catching up, as we usually do, recounting the events of the day as I mindlessly prepared dinner, occasionally pausing our conversation to answer one of our four-year-old daughter's constant questions, or tending to the needs of our then seventeen-month-old son. At this point in life, my priorities included my two children, my husband, and my job. Especially at the end of these long days, I typically didn't have energy left over to dedicate to anything else. On this night, however, my mother told me something that would spark a fire in me that, to this day, has only grown to blaze hotter, brighter, and with more passion than I ever knew I had.

"Did you hear about the law they passed in New York yesterday?" my mother asked. As it had been another busy day in my own isolated world, I responded that I hadn't. "I just heard on the news today," she said, "that they passed a law that would allow a baby to be aborted through all nine months of pregnancy, for any reason." She was referencing the Reproductive Health Act (RHA), signed into law by Governor Andrew Cuomo in New York on January 22, 2019, which indeed, effectively said just that. My mind started spinning in disbelief, and for me in that moment, something clicked in a way that, for some reason, it never had before. Time stood still. "That can't be true," I said matter-of-factly. All of a sudden, the thought of my precious tiny patients being killed in an abortion procedure gripped my heart and mind—a thought that paralyzed me. And in that moment, the reality of abortion overwhelmed me in a way I had never before experienced.

I could not sleep that night, or the night after. I could not reconcile this law taking effect in a state neighboring the one in which I practice medicine. It hit so close to home, from medical, ethical, spiritual, and personal standpoints. Although this was not the first state to pass such a piece of legislation, it was one of the most widely publicized decisions in recent times, even resulting in the Empire State Building being lit up in pink to celebrate this grisly "accomplishment," and was the first one to catch the attention of the public eye in such a dramatic way.

The media worked feverishly in the days and weeks to follow to defend this gruesome piece of legislation, rushing to explain that these "late-term" or post-viability abortions after about 20 weeks of pregnancy would only happen in cases when the health of the mother was in danger. This law would only apply, we were told, in cases when abortion was necessary "to protect the patient's life or health," or in the case of a mother carrying a "non-viable" baby.[1] These were the parameters, couched as they were in ambiguous language yet extrapolated to include the emotional, social, or financial health of the mother, so that it effectively legalized abortion at any time for any reason. As explained by New York State Senator Liz Krueger, "The RHA legalizes abortion after 24 weeks of pregnancy if a woman's health is at risk. . . . in consultation with the pregnant woman, a medical provider determines whether her health is at risk, exercising medical judgment upon considering a variety of factors. One of many factors considered is the woman's *mental health*."[2] The consideration of "mental health" is so broad and nonspecific that it could easily be used as justification in any case where an abortion is requested.

NARAL Pro-choice America's website provides an equally vague and ever-pliable explanation: "New York allows women eligible for state medical assistance for general health care to obtain public funds to pay for medically necessary abortion services. 'Medically necessary' is defined as necessary to prevent, diagnose, correct, or cure conditions in the person that cause *acute suffering*, endanger life, result in illness or infirmity, *interfere with a person's capacity for normal activity*, or threaten some significant handicap."[3] These criteria are quite ambiguous and leave an enormous amount of room for interpretation and debate, to the point where almost any case could be considered "medically necessary." After all, any woman who has given birth knows that the process of delivering a child causes some degree of "acute suffering." Even simply raising a child could be said to "interfere with a person's capacity for normal activity," as every new parent comes to understand. These criteria and justifications essentially allow for abortion on demand, at any time, and for any reason.

Is Abortion Ever Really Necessary?

Despite the best arguments of politicians and the media, the statistics on abortion fly in the face of attempts to rationalize these new laws. The Guttmacher Institute, which reports on abortion surveillance statistics, shows that the overwhelming majority of late-term abortions occur for the same reasons that mothers normally seek abortions in the first trimester, and thus have nothing to do with medical concerns for either the mother or baby.[4] As explained by James Studnicki, from the Charlotte Lozier Institute:

> While the occasional politician or news reporter will still indicate that late-term abortions are most often performed in

> the case of "severe fetal anomalies" or to "save the woman's life," the trajectory of the peer-reviewed research literature has been obvious for decades: most late-term abortions are elective, done on healthy women with healthy fetuses, and for the same reasons given by women experiencing first trimester abortions. The Guttmacher Institute has provided a number of reports over 2 decades which have identified the reasons why women choose abortion, and they have consistently reported that childbearing would interfere with their education, work, and ability to care for existing dependents; would be a financial burden; and would disrupt partner relationships. A more recent Guttmacher study focused on abortion after 20 weeks of gestation and similarly concluded that women seeking late-term abortions were not doing so for reasons of fetal anomaly or life endangerment. The study further concluded that late-term abortion seekers were younger and more likely to be unemployed than those seeking earlier abortions.[5]

Thus, the arguments of lawmakers and the media are *statistically misleading*. Furthermore, they are *scientifically misinformed*, as abortion is never necessary to preserve the health or life of the mother. There are certainly a variety of serious maternal medical conditions that could negatively impact the length of pregnancy. These include dangerously high blood pressure (called *preeclampsia*), life-threatening diabetes, cancer, decompensating heart disease, and a number of other very serious medical conditions. My entire career has been dedicated to helping the children of women who suffer from these serious and life-threatening, pregnancy-related illnesses. And when a maternal condition linked to pregnancy imminently jeopardizes a mother's health or life, her pregnancy must end. However, it is *never* necessary for the pregnancy to end in an abortion, which intentionally ends the life of the child. What these mothers require is a *preterm delivery*, not abortion. There are numerous reasons this is so.

Before the child is capable of surviving outside the womb (a time referred to as *viability*), at around 22 to 24 weeks of gestational age, every effort should be made to treat the mother's condition and safely prolong the pregnancy, as long as the mother's life and health is not imminently in danger. Very rarely, however, best efforts to treat the mother's condition while safely prolonging the pregnancy may be unsuccessful, and in these cases, a previable separation of the mother and the child may become necessary. As explained by Dr. Donna Harrison, Executive Director of the American Academy of Prolife OB/GYNs (AAPLOG):

> There will be cases when a child is delivered too early to survive outside of the womb in order to save a mother's life. There is a very big difference between previable separations and elective abortion. In these situations where a mother and her fetus must be separated in order to save the life of the mother we would try to optimize the conditions of the separation so that the fetus has the best possibility to live. But there are cases when the baby will not survive the separation due to gestational age. We call these previable separations. These separations are done with the intent to save both if possible, but at least to save the life of one. Previable separations are not the same as elective abortions. The intent of an abortion was made very clear at the Supreme Court hearings over the Partial Birth Abortion Ban. The abortionists argued that the product the abortionist is paid

to produce is a dead baby, and that is what distinguishes a delivery from an abortion. The intent of a delivery is to produce, if possible, both a live baby and live mom. The intent of an abortion is to produce a dead baby.[6]

Past the point of viability, which occurs after about 22 to 24 weeks of gestation (depending on the specific protocols and capabilities of a particular hospital), the child can be delivered either via an induction of labor, or via emergency C-section, depending on the specifics of each case. An emergency C-section is actually a faster method for removing a child from an expectant mother than abortion. An emergency C-section can be completed in less than an hour, whereas an abortion procedure for a 20-week-old fetus takes two to three days to complete due to the cervical dilation process involved. Thus, abortion in these cases would significantly delay treatment and increase a mother's risk of serious complications, including death. It would therefore be medically irresponsible to recommend that a mother with an emergency condition wait two days to have an abortion when an emergency C-section would result in the immediate and safe delivery of the child.

In addition, the current state of modern medicine makes early delivery a very reasonable and responsible manner of caring for the baby. The field of neonatal-perinatal medicine has advanced rapidly over the past decade, such that the limits of survival has been pushed to as young as 22 weeks of gestation, which is also when the majority of life-threatening maternal conditions arise. This has major implications for how pregnancies should be handled in cases of women facing serious illness. For each week that a child is delivered after about 22 weeks, his or her chances of survival outside the womb increase dramatically. In fact, it is universally recommended that children delivered after 25 weeks be fully supported at the time of delivery, as their chances of survival, including survival without disability, are very high—about 90 percent survival for those who receive intensive medical treatment.[7] From my perspective as a physician who regularly interacts with these high-risk mothers and their babies, it is absurd to suggest that protecting the life or health of the mother would ever be used as a justification for abortion after 22 weeks.

Admittedly, some of these babies may ultimately be unable to survive outside the womb. In such cases, they are nevertheless treated with compassion and dignity regardless of the timing of their delivery. Mothers are given the chance to hold and meet their child, and to honor their child's life. Medications can be administered to the baby as needed in order to alleviate suffering or pain if they are unable to benefit from medical technology and unable to survive outside the womb due to extreme prematurity or another condition. It is appropriate to briefly mention here the concept of fetal pain, which is another significant issue in the abortion debate, as there is ample scientific evidence to support the fact that babies feel pain in the womb as early as 14 weeks of gestation, adding further significance to the horrific injustice of abortion.[8]

Many babies, however, who are labeled as "non-viable" and subsequently encouraged to be aborted would be more appropriately described as having a "life-limiting condition," which is any condition likely to shorten the child's life expectancy. It can be very difficult to predict the exact amount of time that any given child with one of these life-limiting conditions will survive outside the womb, which is why this term is now preferred to the term "non-viable." The list of qualifying conditions is too long to list in this setting but includes a number of major genetic anomalies (such as

Trisomy 13 and 18) and various major organ abnormalities (such as bilateral renal agenesis, pulmonary hypoplasia, various complex cardiac anomalies, anencephaly, among others). Some children with such life-limiting conditions will survive much longer than anticipated—especially in the cases of children born with various genetic anomalies—and often they have a better "quality of life" than predicted by physicians. Studies have found that physicians frequently underestimate the quality of life for children born with various life-limiting conditions, as compared to the quality of life reported by the children's parents.[9] Delivery and subsequent enrollment into a neonatal palliative care program—similar to adult hospice but with a broader scope and view in order to exist alongside curative interventions when appropriate—is available to mothers who are carrying babies with these life-limiting conditions.

To give a few more examples, it is helpful to discuss two specific medical conditions arising during pregnancy that some physicians have attempted to use as justification for abortion. In an article published in 2019 by *Science Feedback*, two pro-abortion physicians, Drs. Dan Grossman and Robyn Shickler, attempted to refute the claim that abortion is never medically necessary by claiming, "Certain medical conditions such as placenta previa and HELLP syndrome can make abortion a necessary medical procedure in order to prevent the mother's death."[10] AAPLOG Chairman of the Board, Dr. Christina Francis, directly responds to these two particular justifications for abortion, explaining:

> Placenta previa is a condition in which the placenta covers the cervix, making a vaginal delivery impossible due to the possibility of life-threatening hemorrhage if labor occurs. These are frequently diagnosed in pregnancy on ultrasound

around 20 weeks; however approximately 90% of these will resolve on their own before delivery. If significant hemorrhage occurs due to a placenta previa (which again is so rare prior to viability that no incidence is even reported), the patient should be taken for an emergency C-section which is the most expedient way to get her bleeding under control. It would be medically dangerous and irresponsible to try to do an abortion since any instrumentation through the cervix would pierce the placenta and cause immediate massive bleeding. An abortion would take significantly longer in this case and be much riskier for the mother.

Secondly, the incidence of pre-eclampsia with severe features and/or HELLP syndrome prior to viability is exceedingly rare. Per the Society of Maternal Fetal Medicine, the incidence of severe pre-eclampsia prior to 34 weeks is only 0.3% of all pregnancies (incidence of HELLP syndrome would be significantly lower). Prior to 22–24 weeks the incidence is significantly lower. It is not the common situation in the pre-viable period that Drs. Grossman and Shickler would like people to believe. When HELLP syndrome does occur, it necessitates early delivery—not an abortion. In this situation, separation of the mother and fetus can occur in a way that respects the dignity of both of their lives, and if possible, save both."[11]

As powerfully illustrated by the above two cases, it is important to understand that a single medical condition can sometimes be handled in two very different ways. The approach taken can depend entirely on the physician's attitudes and beliefs regarding the value of human life. As a practicing physician, sadly, I see this discrepancy often. Physicians who do not particularly value each human life will seek justifications for abortion, and/or may not fight as hard to save an individual patient (particularly in the case of a baby born around the limits of viability or with a life-limiting condition). On the other hand, physicians who do indeed value each human life at each stage will do everything within their power to promote the life and health of both the mother and her child. An individual physician's attitude and beliefs often directly impact patient care, literally proving to be the difference between life and death in too many cases.

It is also important to discuss the relatively rare situation known as an *ectopic pregnancy*. This is when a preborn child implants in the mother's fallopian tube (most commonly) or somewhere outside the uterus, both of which are hostile environments for supporting the preborn child's continued development. Unfortunately, because a preborn child cannot continue to grow and develop anywhere other than the mother's uterus prior to 21 to 22 weeks of gestation, these pregnancies will inevitably end in a miscarriage. Sadly, in these circumstances, the preborn child must be removed from the fallopian tube, as the inevitable miscarriage may indeed cause the fallopian tube to rupture, resulting in a life-threatening hemorrhage. These procedures, however, are not, and have never been, considered abortions and should not be confused as such, as the intent is not to kill the child, but rather to save the mother's life in the management of an inevitable miscarriage. *Indeed, there is not a single maternal or fetal condition that necessitates that an abortion procedure be performed, whose purpose is directly and intentionally to end the life of a preborn child.*

My perspective on these matters is neither new nor unique. Over a thousand experienced physicians around the world confirm, in a document known as "The Dublin Declaration," that there is not a single maternal medical condition that necessitates an abortion. This document states,

> As experienced practitioners and researchers in obstetrics and gynaecology, we affirm that direct abortion—the purposeful destruction of the unborn child—is not medically necessary to save the life of a woman.
>
> We uphold that there is a fundamental difference between abortion, and necessary medical treatments that are carried out to save the life of the mother, even if such treatment results in the loss of life of her unborn child.
>
> We confirm that the prohibition of abortion does not affect, in any way, the availability of optimal care to pregnant women.[12]

In summary, early delivery is *always* an option in order to protect the mother if and when her health or life is truly in jeopardy.

The Great Deception of Abortion

Until I started seeing the issue of abortion through a spiritual lens, it was difficult for me to understand how other physicians could be blind to the reality that abortion is always murder and is never medically necessary. The Bible tells us clearly that Satan is the father of lies, that he has been murdering from the beginning, and that those who do evil are carrying out his desires (John 8:44). Once I reflected on this, it became clear to me that some indeed use medical jargon and deceptive medical arguments to cover up this profoundly immoral practice. After all, if it were clearly shown that abortion was in fact "medically necessary to save a mother's life," it would be more difficult to insist that killing preborn children should be illegal.

We, however, have been created by a loving God, who is wise beyond our incredibly finite understanding and has expertly designed a safe home for vulnerable human beings to grow—the womb: a sacred place which was never intended to become a battleground between a mother and her child. Although not every child is able to stay in this protective, nurturing environment for all nine months, and some children do need to be delivered early, there is absolutely no maternal medical condition which requires the murder of preborn children.

It is my prayer that the Lord would take off the veil that has blinded and deceived so many even in the medical community, allowing them either to remain silent on this mass genocide, or to actively support it. Ultimately, it is a spiritual battle and must be fought not only with sound logic and reason, but with prayer. Many in the medical profession are intelligent enough to understand that abortion ends the life of another human being, but this alone is not enough to change their minds. All the facts, logic, statistics, and medical research in the world are, unfortunately, not enough to convince them of the immorality and injustice of abortion. The hearts and minds of many on the pro-choice side will not be changed by rational, science-based arguments alone. What is needed is the power of Christ, who is able to "do immeasurably more than all we ask or imagine, according to his power that is at work within us" (Eph. 3:20 NIV). If we rely solely on appeals to science and statistics, we will fail to change their hearts and minds because, in many cases, this is a spiritual battle and must be fought accordingly.

An important perspective to include on this point is the powerful testimony of former abortionist Dr. David Brewer, who became a believer in Christ and now devotes his life to the pro-life cause. His story illustrates how those in the medical community can become deceived, calloused, and blinded to the immoral and unnecessary practice of abortion. He opens his story by describing how his journey to become an abortionist began:

> It happened after medical school as I began my residency in OB/GYN. I can vividly remember that day. I remember watching the resident doctor sitting down and putting the tube in and removing the contents. I saw the bloody material sucked down the plastic tube and it went into a big jar. The first abortion I had ever witnessed; I had no idea what to expect.
>
> It was my job after the abortion had taken place to go see what was inside of that big jar. It was kind of neat, learning another procedure. I wasn't a Christian; I didn't have any views on abortion; I was in a training program; this was a brand-new experience. As I opened the jar and took out the little piece of stockinette the resident doctor said, "Now open it and put it on that blue towel and check it out. We want to make sure that we got it all." I thought; Oh, that will be exciting—hands-on experience, looking at tissue. I opened the sock up and I put it on the towel and there were the parts of a little person. I'd taken anatomy; I was a medical student; I knew what I was looking at. There was a little scapula and some ribs and then I saw a little hand and the arms. It was terrible, it was like somebody put a hot poker into me.
>
> I checked it out and there were two arms, two legs, a head, etc., and I turned and said, "I guess you got it all." That was a very hard experience for me to go through

emotionally. If I'd been a Christian it would have been simple—I wouldn't have been there. But there I was—with no real convictions. So how did I handle this abortion issue? I did what a lot of us do throughout our lives, we don't do anything. I didn't talk with anybody about it. I didn't talk with my folks about it. I didn't think about it. I did nothing.[13]

As an experienced OB-GYN who also knew firsthand that abortion is never medically necessary but is instead electively requested, Brewer continued to perform abortions, suppressing his guilt in order to justify his actions. He even details his participation in the C-section and hysterectomy of a woman four or five months pregnant, which resulted in the needless death of her baby:

I remember as we made the incision in the uterus, to see the baby move underneath the sack of membranes as the Caesarian incision was made before the doctor broke the water. The thought came to me, my God, that's a person!

At that instant he broke the water and I had that terrible pain in my heart. He delivered the baby and I couldn't even touch it. I wasn't much of an assistant; I just stood there and the reality of what was going on finally began to seep in to my callused brain and heart. We simply took that little baby that was making little sounds and was moving and kicking and set it on the table in a cold stainless steel bowl. Every time I would look over, while we were repairing the incision in the uterus, I would see that little person kicking and moving in that bowl. It kicked and moved less and less as time went on. I can remember going over and looking at that baby when we were done with surgery and the baby

> was still alive. You could see the chest moving as the heart beat and the baby would try and take a little breath.

That day and that experience should have been enough to stop Dr. Brewer from continuing to participate in the murder of vulnerable human beings. And yet he continued performing abortions, establishing new intellectual barriers along the way to safeguard his conscience. He explains:

> What do we do when something really hurts us? We either stand up to it or we run. I wasn't equipped to stand up, and so I ran. The way I ran was by putting up barriers. In my mind, I decided that life began when a baby could survive outside the uterus. . . . That meant that the hysterotomy that I helped on was not an abortion because the baby couldn't have survived outside. After all, it sat in the dish and died. . . .
>
> Then I saw more babies being born earlier and earlier with the advances in our neonatal intensive care units. As the technology increased, suddenly they were having luck with babies that were 28 weeks old, and then 27 weeks, and then 26 weeks. So my barriers began to crumble. . . . Then I got to thinking maybe it's 20 weeks. No wait, it's a baby when it's all formed, so I began thinking after 12 weeks! All I was doing was avoiding the truth. . . .
>
> And once I made that startling discovery, it was very simple for me to stop doing abortions.

As Dr. Brewer's testimony shows, abortion is approved and practiced when hearts become hardened and truth is ignored. Satan is indeed the father of lies, and it is because of his deceit that murder and evil are encouraged and continue (John 8:44).

We must therefore pray that those in the medical field, who already know the scientific facts about abortion, who cannot be won over by logically sound arguments, will have their eyes opened and hearts softened by Christ, so that they too will be able to accept the truth that they ultimately and already know deep down. We must pray that women who have believed the lie that their abortion was "medically necessary" will have their hearts softened and will ultimately come to a place of healing and restoration by accepting the forgiveness and grace available through faith in Jesus Christ. We must also pray that those in the community who are deceived by pro-choice arguments will come to know the truth, and that the truth will inspire them to do what they can to protect preborn children.

From the NICU to a New Family

The needlessness of abortion can be illustrated through a simple story. It is the story of a young, single mother of three, pregnant again—already struggling to care well for her three other children. This time, however, her pregnancy was somehow concealed and unknown even to herself. At about what was later realized to be her 24th week of pregnancy, the woman began to feel a strong, overwhelming, though familiar pain—the pain of childbirth. She was rushed to the hospital where she delivered her son, who emerged limp, lifeless, and without a heartbeat. He arrived the same way an aborted baby emerges from the womb, except intact.

One might assume that an unresponsive child born so prematurely would have no chance of survival. Yet a skilled nurse practitioner was ready for his delivery, at which time she inserted a breathing tube, administered CPR, and gave him multiple doses of a heart-restarting medication. After ten minutes of vigorous resuscitation, the baby boy's heart started beating again. All of these heroic measures were taken for a child whom many in our society would have said has little to no chance of living—worse yet, has little to no value. This child, whom many in our society would have said was a valid abortion candidate so as not to become a burden for his mother, came back to life.

The newborn first grew and developed inside a heated incubator in the NICU, initially sustained by a breathing tube connected to a ventilator. Meanwhile, a few states away, a young childless married couple was anxiously waiting their turn to adopt. Little did they know their son-to-be had just entered into the world in this incredible way.

Only a few days after his dramatic delivery, the boy's adoptive parents came to meet him for the first time in the NICU, with tears of joy in their eyes. He was the answer to their prayers. They did not leave his side. He was their treasured son, their new pride and joy, whom they watched and sat beside each day as he continued to fight for his own life. He eventually grew strong enough to leave the NICU, go home with his new parents, and live his life. The child, whom society would have said was worthless, became the family's greatest treasure. He went from being a potential "burden" to his young, single, overwhelmed mother, to becoming the joy of his adoptive mother and father, who cuddled, kissed, and doted on him at every opportunity. His adoptive parents will tell you that he is here for a reason, because every child is.

Conclusion

Is abortion ever medically necessary? No, it isn't. Not in the first trimester, not in the second trimester, not in the third trimester. Never. Plain and simple. There is always a life-affirming answer to every complex and serious medical concern arising in pregnancy. We must pray that God will open our country's eyes in a profound way to see clearly the deception used to justify abortion, so that no child is ever murdered in the womb. Never again.

CLAIM 6

Abortions Are Helpful to Women and Society

16

The Truth about Post-Abortive Trauma: The Personal Account of a Survivor and Activist

—Victoria Robinson—

Discussing the effects of abortion is challenging because post-abortive individuals have not been sufficiently researched. Much of the research that does exist is contested, heavily politicized, and does not account for the experiences of many who have received abortions.[1] And the latter is understandable because, who would want to be a case study? Admitting to an abortion is very difficult for the post-abortive mother or father. The guilt, shame, and regret are too painful. Being reminded of, much less speaking about, a past abortion is very difficult. For many, it is easier to bury the past than to speak about it.

I know this all too well. I know because abortion is a part of my past as well. I am a woman who once chose abortion, and this choice has deeply affected my own life. Not only that, I have met or counseled thousands of other post-abortive women and men in my twenty-three-year career in the pro-life movement, not only in this country but throughout the world.

My Abortion Story

Thirty-three years—396 months—12,045 days. That's how long it has been since I made the decision to drive myself to an abortion clinic in Charlotte, North Carolina, to end the life of my eight-week-old unborn baby. I was already a mother of two little girls (two and four years old), so it wasn't as though I was unaware of the outcome of a pregnancy. I knew. But when you find yourself in a crisis, you hear what you think you need to hear and do what you think you need to do. You just want the crisis to go away.

I was a young, single mother when my then-husband decided he didn't want to be married to me any longer. He left. We lived in North Carolina and he moved to California—he couldn't have gone farther away from us. Without any emotional or financial support from him, I found myself in one of the most desperate situations of my life. I had two very young daughters who were looking to their very broken mother for answers. And I just didn't have them. My self-esteem was shot to pieces, my self-worth nonexistent, and my bank account empty.

I ended up taking a job at a health club, working up to fourteen hours a day, just to put food on the table. It should come as no surprise that this young, lonely, vulnerable, broken woman would find herself in an unhealthy relationship nine months later. He said all the right words and paid all the necessary attention. I was willing to do anything for him, including killing my child.

When I told him I was pregnant, I didn't receive the celebratory response I had hoped for and believed he would provide. Instead, the man I loved and was so sure I would spend the rest of my life with was shocked. Then he became incredibly convincing. I was already a mess, asking myself how I could have let this happen, so it was easy for him to manipulate this naïve young mother into believing what was best.

After encouraging me to call the abortion clinic in Charlotte, my boyfriend soon realized he had found an ally in the kind woman on the other end of the line. She, too, agreed wholeheartedly with him about what had to be done. And she was just as convincing.

After sharing my situation and concerns, she compassionately told me she understood exactly what I was going through. Knowing my financial struggles as a single mother, she told me, "Don't you think it would be very selfish of you to bring another mouth to feed when you can barely take care of the two you already have? Besides, you're so early, there's nothing there. We'll get you in right away and take care of it. It will be no more than like having a tumor removed." By the time we hung up, I had an appointment for three days later on a Saturday morning.

Over the course of those three days, I agonized over the decision. I cried, got a grip, then cried again. I hired a babysitter to take care of my two young daughters, and when Saturday morning came, I was driving myself to an abortion clinic thirty minutes away, crying and begging this "tumor" for forgiveness.

On that morning, the abortion clinic took my baby. But they were never able to take the *memory* of my baby.

After my abortion, I thought I would never be the same again. The emotional toll of making such a choice was more than I could bear. Physically, I began to experience what I now know as anxiety attacks. Before, I wasn't one who dreamed a lot. After my abortion, I started having nightmares about that day. In my dream, I ran out, but then I would wake up and realize it wasn't real. I would lay my hand over my stomach as if my child was still there, full well knowing my child was gone and my womb was empty. Quite often, I would ask myself how I would ever be normal again. I was convinced I looked different and others could see right through my fake smile. I became a shell of a person; I was numb. Each day that I got out of bed, I was just going through the motions. I resolved myself to this new life and I knew I deserved nothing less for what I had done.

It wasn't until over a decade later, after years of being involved in abusive relationships and self-destructive behaviors, I realized there was help available to me as a post-abortive woman. It was a pregnancy resource center that offered help to me, without condemnation or judgment. The help they gave not only healed my wounds, but it set me on a course and connected me to a cause I'm passionate about to this day.

My Post-Abortive Ministry

When I first entered the world of pro-life advocacy, I began as a volunteer at the local pregnancy resource center (PRC) in Concord, North Carolina, where after seven years I became the executive director. PRCs are in every major city of the country and are the alternative to—in fact, the complete opposite of—abortion clinics. They are nonprofit organizations funded by churches, individuals, and businesses that provide pregnancy tests, STD testing, ultrasound, maternity clothing, baby supplies, parenting classes, education, and pregnancy-decision counseling—all free of charge—with the goal of safeguarding the health of the mother and the success of her pregnancy.

At the Concord PRC, my responsibilities did not stop with running the operations. I was also a trained counselor. More times than I can count, I counseled women who were contemplating abortion, and also those who had already chosen abortion.

For example, women who had already scheduled an abortion would often come for an ultrasound appointment. The ultrasound would show the mom the age and size of her unborn child, which was necessary for estimating the cost of her abortion—the further along her pregnancy, the higher the cost.

One of my favorite parts of the job was being in the ultrasound room with these clients. It was always a marvel to witness their reactions as they saw their unborn child for the first time. Countless of these women who already had abortions scheduled were in awe of how *human* their baby looked. Imagine their shock and surprise to see their child moving around in their womb after being told by the abortion clinic worker they were only carrying a "blob of tissue" or "clump of cells." I was there when these women wept and realized, "That's my baby." Nine out of ten times, after our nurse performed the free ultrasound, these women who had already decided to abort, changed their minds after seeing their babies. I cancelled many of their abortion appointments myself, at their request. It was difficult for them to deny a heartbeat, arms, or legs.

I held the hands of these women as they were inconsolable with the realization of what they had almost done, and in some cases what they did do. I counseled one young woman for three weeks. Her mother and boyfriend were pressuring her to have an abortion, but she had already seen her fourteen-week baby on an ultrasound and was determined to carry her child to full-term. Sadly, the pressure from her own mother eventually became too great and she succumbed to abortion. Afterward, she came to me begging, "Get my baby back!" She sobbed as she cried, "Why didn't I listen to you? What have I done?"

I could tell you thousands of heart-wrenching stories just like this one. These are real people who are now living with real scars, due to abortion. Once they came to the realization their abortion was a permanent reaction to a temporary problem, they were broken.

I saw the need for this kind of post-abortion counseling decades ago. Not only the need in my own life, but in the lives of so many women I came into contact with. That is when I decided to start a nonprofit that would focus on post-abortion healing. I founded an organization called Re-Assemble, dedicated to counseling post-abortive men and women around the country, and to educating the public on the damaging effects of abortion. The need is great. Through Re-Assemble, I have been facilitating abortion recovery weekend retreats for over fifteen years. To this day, I have a waiting list.

I have been on the front lines of the abortion issue for over two decades, as a counselor, educator, and public speaker. Not only did I myself choose abortion over thirty-three years ago (still more on that later), but through my work with PRCs and Re-Assemble, I have also met and worked with thousands of women and men who have their own abortion stories to tell.

The Effects of Abortion on Women

The traumatic effects of abortion do not discriminate between sex or circumstances. For the post-abortive woman, it doesn't matter how she came to the decision. Whether she was talked into an abortion, pressured into an abortion, forced into an abortion, or chose to have an abortion on her own accord, it doesn't matter. The same goes for the post-abortive man, about whom we'll talk below. Whether he paid for the abortion, pressured his girlfriend into an abortion, forced his wife into an abortion, or only learned about it after the fact—it doesn't matter. Their heartbreak is real.

The majority of women who choose abortion do not come out unscathed. The same woman who walks into an abortion clinic is not the same woman who walks out. Many of the women who choose abortion suffer from physical, emotional, and psychological effects. Some women will suffer from immediate physical complications—ranging from mild pain to moderate or severe injury, such as hemorrhaging, infection, or sepsis—while others will experience long-term health or pregnancy challenges—such as miscarriage, infertility, or disease.[2] Some women will experience only (or also) emotional trauma, such as anxiety, guilt, or depression.[3] Often, these women will begin showing signs of trauma immediately following the procedure. For others, however, it could be months or years before the symptoms surface, and for still others, their wounds won't show for decades.

Here is a list of just some of the more common emotional issues faced by the post-abortive woman: *heartbreak, guilt, shame, low self-esteem, regret, fear of losing a living child, fear of never getting pregnant again, substance abuse, alcoholism, cutting, self-destructive relationships, abusive relationships, promiscuity, numbness, problems connecting with others, isolation, destroying healthy relationships, becoming a helicopter mom.*[4]

Women who later become pregnant with a wanted child experience incredible anxiety about losing the pregnancy as some sort of divine retribution for having had an abortion. In return, their future pregnancies are filled with fear, rather than joy.

Once they do have kids, many post-abortive mothers become

"helicopter moms," fearful that something will happen to their child or children. Their children become confused when mommy doesn't allow them to play with friends or go anywhere without them anymore.

Many post-abortive women bury their pain for years before seeking out help. It is easier for them to try to forget the abortion ever happened than it is to deal with the ramifications of the decision. The majority of post-abortive women don't realize that some of the harmful, destructive behaviors they engage in stem from a past abortion. They will find themselves confused and wonder why they are so angry. Post-abortive women are convinced they don't deserve to be happy and quite frequently they find themselves sabotaging healthy relationships.

Post-abortive women also find themselves drawn to abusive men because, subconsciously, they believe they deserve the abuse. They have convinced themselves and others they don't deserve to be happy for what they have done.

Many post-abortive women believe the lie they aren't allowed to grieve the loss of their child since the child died by their own hand. I once met a woman in her sixties (I'll call her Brenda) who told me she didn't know she was allowed to grieve. I had just finished speaking at a fundraising event for a local Pregnancy Resource Center in Wyoming when Brenda approached me. I could tell she had been crying. She pulled me aside and said, "I didn't know what this event was about tonight. My friend asked me to come last minute. When I heard you speak about aborting your child, I was shocked. When I heard you say you grieve, I was confused. And when I heard you talk about the help you received, I was hopeful." She continued, "I didn't know women like you and me were allowed to grieve, and I didn't know there was any help available for people like me. Thank you for giving me permission to grieve and please tell me where to go for help." Brenda had chosen abortion forty-two years prior to that evening and it had haunted her to that day. As Brenda and I parted ways, I hugged her. I told her I was so sorry for her loss. She answered, "Losses. You mean you're sorry for my losses. I was carrying twins."

You may be thinking that one person's experience can't constitute millions. That is true. But as I stated earlier, I've been involved in working with post-abortive women for decades. Their experiences are very similar to one another. I've met, counseled, or spoken to thousands of post-abortive parents. I can attest to the pain, guilt, shame, and utter grief they go through. I've seen it, I've smelled it, and I've tasted it. I've lived it myself. And some of their experiences are documented and available for the world to read.[5]

The Effects of Abortion on Men

For too long, we have left men out of the discussion about the effects of abortion. I am determined to change that. When I wrote my book *They Lied to Us,* I called the father of my aborted child. I felt he should know it was about to be published. We had not spoken about our abortion since we broke up. He instantly recognized my voice and began to weep. He told me, "I've been waiting for this call for over a decade. I want to beg your forgiveness." He continued, "I should have protected you and our child. I'm so sorry for what I made you do. Can you forgive me? It's haunted me all these years and I've been in therapy for eight years dealing with it."

At that moment, I realized two things. First, I had not forgiven him completely, which was only hurting myself. Unforgiveness, says the adage, is like taking poison and expecting the other person to die. In that instant, I forgave him. And I felt a new sense of freedom. The second thing I realized was that men are hurting too. That conversation changed the entire trajectory of my work in the pro-life cause. In those precious moments, I knew I could no longer be silent when it came to men and the abortion issue. From that day on, everywhere I speak, whether it is at churches, conferences, or fundraisers, I acknowledge post-abortive fathers. They are just as important and vital to this conversation. These aborted children not only had mothers, but they had fathers as well.

After an abortion, men tend to shy away from commitment. They withdraw from their parents, siblings, friends, and coworkers. They fear getting too close. Others turn to drinking or drugs, or they become workaholics. Most of the time, they don't realize they are doing it. Or, if they do, they don't understand why.

Following is a list of the issues post-abortive men attest they have experienced after being involved in the abortion of their own children: *heartache, guilt, regret, dealing with commitment issues, alcoholism, become workaholics, drug abuse, promiscuity, failure to connect, perfectionists, hard to connect with children, anger issues.*[6]

You'll notice the post-abortive mother and post-abortive father lists have many similarities. That is because each one was a parent on the day they found out about their pregnancy. And each one eventually comes to a point where they can no longer deny the consequences of ending the life of their child. These realizations cause grief and distress for both the mother and the father. Both lose self-esteem and become sure they are unworthy, and doubt that God could ever love or use them. Therefore, they often hide away from the church, or anyone having to do with faith or religion, for fear of being "found out."

Post-abortion recovery is on the rise due to men and women finally speaking out about how an abortion negatively and traumatically transformed their lives. The more abortion is talked about, the more we will see this trend. Nonetheless, the traumatic effects are very real, and avoidable.

Conclusion

Abortion not only destroys a living, breathing human being with its own unique DNA, but it destroys the mothers who choose it. I've counseled thousands of women over my twenty-two-year career—thousands of real-life people who have been traumatized by a decision many were coerced into making by a multibillion-dollar industry that preys on them during the most vulnerable time of their life.

And we can't forget about the men who are struggling as well. Since *Roe v. Wade*, over 62 million abortions have been performed in the United States alone. That's more than 124 million men and women who are "walking wounded." Abortion hurts people. Abortion destroys lives.

Since making the decision to have an abortion, I've gone through my own healing process and have been able to help thousands of others do the same. I've been forgiven and set free from that horrible decision. But the post-abortive man or woman will always long for the child they never knew.

The consequences of abortion to the individual, to families, and to our society as a whole far surpass the challenge of an unplanned pregnancy. It is better for the parent to raise the child or place him or her into adoption than to risk the trauma of abortion.

17

An Expedient Tool: The Harmful Effects of Abortion on Society

—Patrina Mosley—

I once saw a tweet that said, "slavery is job creation." It was meant to convey the silliness of the trending abortion gimmick "abortion is healthcare." I found the tweet very clever because it illustrates that skillful marketing can make anything sound good. The vilest act can be purified and defended if someone is crafty enough to make it sound like an act of virtue.

For example, enslaving an entire race of people as property to be bought, sold, beaten, and raped was once supported in America in the name of "states' rights." The Southern states, ripe with agricultural opportunity, did not want the federal government interfering with their use of slaves. Whether you believe the Civil War was fought over slavery or not, when the North won, one of the outcomes was the abolition of slavery. Would a Southern victory, with their interpretation of "states' rights," have resulted in the same outcome? Probably not.

There is no right to slavery nor to treating a race or subsection of people as being less than human. Abortion is similar to slavery in that it treats people—in this case, children in the womb—as less than human. Like slavery, abortion's supporters justify it under the guise of it being a "right."

Abortion is one of the most brutal forms of violence committed on the human body. The many different methods of abortion include the baby being suctioned out of the mother's womb (aspiration suction)[1] and being physically dismembered (dilation and evacuation, commonly known as dismemberment abortion).[2] In the event of a botched abortion, the unwanted newborn child could be simply left to die or actively put to death by other means (literal infanticide).[3]

Yet the abortion lobby has sanitized all these violent acts by marketing them as "healthcare," "reproductive healthcare," "a women's right to choose," even as an "essential" healthcare service. Amid the 2020–2021 coronavirus pandemic, Michigan Governor Gretchen Whitmer asserted that abortions ought to be deemed essential because they are a "life- sustaining" service.[4] Life sustaining? The very act of elective abortion is to take life, not sustain it. Yet such an act is defended as so-called women's reproductive healthcare.[5]

The first time we see this type of deceptive marketing at work is when Satan approached the woman in the garden of Eden and made disobedience to God sound like an opportunity for enlightenment (Gen. 3:1). How masterful! Adam and Eve could eat from any tree in the garden except from the tree of the knowledge of good and evil. God's command was clear, as was the punishment for disobedience (Gen. 2:17). Yet Satan tricked the woman into desiring something she already had—enlightenment.

Unfortunately, Adam followed his wife in defying God's command. As a result of the first humans' sin, the world faced a myriad of consequences, including the reality of spiritual and physical death. The Bible teaches that rebellion against God is at the very core of all sin, yet the "father of lies" appeared as an "angel of light" (John 8:44; 2 Cor. 11:13–15) and managed to advertise disobedience as an opportunity for enlightenment. In retrospect, Eve was "enlightened" after eating the forbidden fruit, but it did not lead to true flourishing. Rather, it led to much hurt and pain for her and the rest of the human race.

Had Adam and Eve remained in their innocence and rejected Satan's crafty attempts to convince them that evil was good, who knows what bliss we humans might have enjoyed. Prior to Adam and Eve's fall into sin, they enjoyed direct fellowship with God! Now, because of their actions, death has entered the world, and all humans have a sinful nature (Rom. 5:12). Humanity is spiritually separated from God and held accountable by Him for our sins.

However, God is merciful. Before time began, He already had a plan to redeem humankind from the rebellion initiated by Adam and Eve (Col. 1:15–20; Rev. 13:8). In Romans 6:23, the apostle Paul tells us that the wages we earn from our sin is death, but that the gift of God is eternal life through His Son, Jesus Christ. Christ willingly became our substitute to take the punishment of God; whoever repents and places their trust in Christ will have eternal life. This is the gospel message, and its promises are true, including for those who have had abortions or played a role in an abortion. The gospel is the cure for both our souls and our society.

Although the gospel offers hope for sinners, Satan is still at work in the world. One of God's most straightforward commands is "You shall not murder" (Ex. 20:13 NIV). As we can see in the Bible, the ancients believed that life begins in the womb, even though they were without the benefit of ultrasound technology (Ps. 139:13–16). Yet today, the taking of life in the womb has been dressed up as "a woman's choice."

You cannot market abortion as something "good" and expect society to flourish. The repercussions of abortion have led to psychological and emotional damage to women and men alike, while having far-reaching consequences beyond individual lives. This chapter will analyze abortion's debilitating effects on men, women, and greater society, demonstrating that even as abortion is touted as a tool for accomplishing good, it is in reality nothing short of an expedient tool producing evil.

Harmful Effects on Women

The abortion industry advertises its services as the gateway to freedom and empowerment that the woman is otherwise lacking. All she has to do in exchange is reject and despise her natural inclination to nurture. The truth is, a woman's unique ability to give life to the world *is* empowerment, and her freedom to choose can come in the choice of whom she will share that power of procreation with, in holy matrimony. Does the false promise of "freedom" and "empowerment" sound familiar, once again deceiving the woman to desire something she already has (Gen. 3:6)?

The result of this "exchange" of truth for lies has been traumatic. While abortion takes a child's life away, it does not change the fact that the woman was once a mother. The trauma of this cannot be understated, and many women suffer in silence with this secret because they see no room for them within the "empowered women" narrative. For some women, the trauma is so devastating that they attempt to cope with drugs, alcohol, suicide, and other risky behaviors.[6] Other women, the ones who get the spotlight and a microphone, are those who choose to cope by way of bitter defiance, as if taking the life of their child was necessary to prove something. Proverbs 14:10 (NIV) says, "Each heart knows its own bitterness, and no one else can share its joy," but Psalm 44:21 tells us that God knows the secrets of our hearts. We may not know, but God knows. So when we see celebrities and brash, outspoken abortion advocates angrily push abortion rights or "shout their abortion," we should pray for them. Who knows what they are dealing with in their hearts? Perhaps this is the way they choose to cope. Pray they turn to God who can heal them of all brokenness and pain, giving them a clean slate to start a new life in Him (2 Cor. 5:17).

According to the latest data, one in four women undergo abortion in the United States, and over half of abortions are committed by women who claim a religious affiliation.[7] Knowing this, we must acknowledge that abortion has produced many broken women in our society, and many of them could be sitting in the pews of our churches. We have an incredible opportunity to minister to these women, and we must be intentional about hearing their stories and ministering to their needs.

A very insightful study was done on post-abortive women and their decision to abort.[8] The respondents were mostly older women looking back at their decision to abort when they were in their twenties or thirties. Their answers reveal how their "choice" to pursue abortion still affects them many years later. Very few spoke of feeling "empowered," like so many contemporary feminists maintain. Instead, the nearly 1,000 women participating in the study reported carrying a toxic mix of negative emotions. Nearly 32 percent of these women expressed no positives from their abortion experience, except that for some it led to finding faith in Christ or participating in pro-life advocacy as a result of their abortion experience.

For years, abortion surveillance reports have shown that most women seek an abortion between the ages of 20 and 34,[9] typically the season of life when one is pursuing education or careers. Feminist rhetoric celebrates the narrative that "women can have it all," while also celebrating a woman terminating the life of her child in her efforts to achieve success. What does abortion give to the mother in exchange for the life of her child? If a woman has to choose abortion to get ahead, that means something is wrong with the priorities of our society, and those who support "abortion as freedom" and "you can have it all" narratives are lying—apparently the choice is either/or.

In the same survey, over 70 percent of the women said their decision to abort included subtle pressure; nearly 60 percent said they did it to make others happy. Abortion does not help women; it only makes things easier for people around them—like a boss, partner, potential caretakers, and others. Telling a woman she can have it *all* by simply eliminating part of the "all" (i.e., her child) is a tragic contradiction. No matter how many awards or accolades one can get from popular culture, they will never replace the child that was denied life.

Satan deceives women into thinking they cannot handle the pregnancy or that they have a God-given right to convenience and ease. Although some women deceptively couch their "abortion freedom" in spiritual language (e.g., "thank God I have this right"), the truth is found in Proverbs 3:5–6, which says, "Trust in the LORD with all your heart and lean not on your own understanding; in all your ways submit to him, and he will make your paths straight" (NIV). The truth is that women *can* have it all, just maybe not all at the same time. But by placing our trust in God and allowing His Word to guide us, we will find our way to a fruitful life, and God will guard our path by the loving care and strength He has already prepared to give us. Earthly accolades will fade away. God's Word and care will not.

In this country, abortions can be financially costly.[10] But the emotional, mental, and spiritual costs are much higher. Abortionists promise a quick fix to the problem of an unplanned pregnancy but fail to mention that the transaction often includes the possibility of bodily damage, grief, anger, depression, anxiety, sleepless nights, substance abuse, and emotional isolation. The "empowered" mob will not be there to ease these adverse effects, nor do they have the ability to do so. Only Christ gives true peace, and it costs us nothing, and Him everything on the cross.

Harmful Effects on Men

For men, abortion can function as an escape hatch within sexual encounters. Men no longer must take responsibility for the consequences of sex and have been told by modern culture that they have no say in whether the child he helped create should live or die. By today's standard, to be truly "woke" as a man is to forsake their God-given duty to lead and protect. Progressive voices in our culture now tell men that in order for them to be considered "pro-woman," they must abolish their "patriarchal oppression" by submitting to ambivalence for the woman, their child, and their future. How backwards does this sound? Now, of course, this nonsense all goes out the window when child-support or alimony is considered. According to the "woke," it is only after the child is born that the man has a responsibility to care for his child. But according to God's Word, which affirms the personhood of the unborn, a man's responsibility to his child begins at the moment that child exists—at the moment of conception.

For the men who do not want to answer the call of responsibility, the hook-up culture and abortion have been great advantages. Sex with no consequences—and no say on the life of the child—equals the opportunity for men to gladly sit back and proclaim with a smirk, "Yeah, down with the patriarchy! This is great!" Men can now indulge their sinful nature as an act of solidarity with the modern woman. This is another deception masterfully constructed by the father of lies.

As mentioned earlier, abortions often come about as a result of outside pressure. Although the majority of abortions are done for the sake of convenience (education, careers, finances), almost half the time it is followed up by relationship problems with partners who are unwilling to become fathers.[11] Men who do not want the woman to continue with the pregnancy have been known to resort to acts of violence against her. We have already seen dozens of news stories of this happening. Intimate partner violence (IPV) occurs so frequently that homicide is the leading cause of death during pregnancy. IPV has become so common that the American College of Obstetricians and Gynecologists (ACOG) has recommended that OBGYNs evaluate whether their patients are experiencing partner support or violence.[12]

Coercive abortion has been a convenient way for sexual abusers to cover up their crimes. It is not unusual for traffickers and pimps to force abortions on their victims and push women back on the streets to find more clients. Women who are trafficked often experience multiple abortions.[13]

However, it should not go unmentioned that many men have

faced regret, shame, and guilt, just as women have, from abortion. Although this is not acknowledged often nor studied to the same extent as it is for women, it should be noted that men have experienced grief due to being silenced in the decision to abort (see chapter 16 of this volume). Grief was a common theme among studies pertaining to men and abortion.[14] These men must cope with the fact that although abortion took their child's life, it did not change the fact that they were once a father. Many men have felt shame for not taking responsibility and sadness for the loss of a child they felt powerless to save.

Harmful Effects on Society

Abortion has become the most expedient tool in high society's attempt to limit the population—primarily of those who are poor, disabled, and people of color. Abortion is rooted in eugenic and Malthusian philosophies, which have been the driving force behind global abortion policies under the guise of "reproductive health."

The belief that overpopulation will deplete natural resources and food supplies has persisted for centuries. Tragically, throughout history, people guided by this belief have argued that limits should be placed on the reproduction of those who would supposedly deplete the most resources—the poor, disabled, and anyone deemed "unfit." This thinking is commonly referred to as Malthusianism, named for political economist Thomas Robert Malthus. Malthusianism laid the foundation for the abortion agenda at work today.[15]

Charles Darwin expounded on Malthus' works with his theory of evolution, which he explained in *On the Origin of Species by Means of Natural Selection, or the Preservation of Favoured Races in the Struggle for Life*.[16] The full, original title of Darwin's book has long been omitted for political reasons. However, Darwin's theory of evolution concluded that there were "lesser races" of people whose breeding should be restricted. The theory of evolution became the foundation for the eugenics movement. In fact, the modern eugenics movement was spearheaded by Darwin's cousin Sir Francis Galton, a scientist who dedicated his work to "the study of agencies under social control that may improve or impair the racial qualities of future generations either physically or mentally."[17] In 1833, Galton coined the term "eugenics," which is rooted in Greek etymology (*eugenês*; cf. 1 Cor. 1:26), meaning "well-born."[18] This philosophy attracted the powerful elites of society and influenced the rollout of abortion on demand.

The nation's leading abortion supplier, Planned Parenthood, was founded by eugenicist Margaret Sanger. As a member of the American Eugenics Society (AES), Sanger dedicated her life's work to solving what she saw as the greatest threat to society, namely, the imbalance of the population between the "fit" and the "unfit."[19] As founder and chief editor of *The Birth Control Review*, Sanger often gave recognition to birth control organizations in foreign countries and the Federation of the Neo-Malthusian Leagues around the world. Sanger's publication featured propaganda targeting women and regular updates on the population control efforts of other countries.

The Ku Klux Klan supported Sanger, and she initiated what she called the "Negro Project." Although Sanger's stated goal was to improve the black community's quality of life, in actuality her project sought to convince Black people to participate in their own demise. Sanger even admitted once, "We do not want the word to go out that we want to exterminate the Negro population."[20]

Incredibly, Sanger's ideas and Planned Parenthood's eugenic

history still guide the organization today. In fact, nearly 80 percent of Planned Parenthood clinics are located within walking distance of African American and Hispanic neighborhoods. Black women receive over 30 percent of all abortions in the United States.[21] African Americans are the nation's slowest growing ethnic group, representing just 12 percent of the population.[22] Is this an interesting coincidence? Hardly. It is the result of decades of racist policies aimed at extinguishing Black and brown babies.

It is worth noting that before changing the organization's name to Planned Parenthood, Sanger's organization was called the American Birth Control League. Changing the name to Planned Parenthood was a strategic attempt to project a more positive image onto their work. Eugenicists came to realize that their ideas would be more accepted if they switched their marketing from telling people that "you are unfit to breed" to getting them to rely on social motivations that would cause them to voluntarily limit their reproduction—such as the fear of having a "defective" child, rearing an "unwanted" child, or economic instability.[23] These fear tactics are skillfully woven into the pattern of abortion. Eugenicists knew that to get women to self-select in limiting their reproduction, there needed to be political bodies at work that would, in the words of Sanger, drive "the whole [population] problem under-ground."[24]

Traces of eugenic ideology can be found in *Roe v. Wade,* the landmark abortion case.[25] The case openly acknowledges that "population growth, pollution, poverty, and racial overtones"[26] factored into the decision. It cites the 1927 *Buck v. Bell* case that legalized involuntary sterilization programs to promote "the welfare of society" and to prevent the nation from "being swamped with incompetence" and would-be criminals.[27] Ruth Bader Ginsburg was even quoted in a *New York Times* interview admitting frankly that she "thought that at the time *Roe* was decided, there was concern about population growth and particularly growth in populations that we don't want to have too many of."[28]

Eugenic ideology has also factored into policy on modern abortion methods. A co-counsel to *Roe* and advisor to Bill Clinton appealed for the approval of the abortifacient drug RU-486, because too many Americans were drawing on the nation's welfare system. In a conversation with President Clinton, the lawyer explained, "You can start immediately to eliminate the barely educated, unhealthy, and poor segment of our country. . . . It's what we all know is true, but we only whisper it."[29]

The Clinton administration steamrolled the approval of "the abortion pill" in 2000. Today, abortions committed by using the pill make up nearly 40 percent of abortions. And in 2019, Gavin Newsom, the Democrat governor of California, signed a bill that will force all public colleges in California to dispense the abortion pill by 2023.[30] This targeting of college students clearly implies that unwanted pregnancies could lead to discontinuing education and result in poverty, and the state would rather pay for mothers to kill their children than to take the chance that these children will become a burden to society. However, nothing has been done to provide more resources to students who are choosing to parent.

The naïve foot-soldiers of abortion advocacy are deceived into thinking that abortion is about a woman's right to choose. In reality, the choice was already made for her by the elite and powerful who understand that abortion is about controlling the population of "those we don't want too many of." Supreme Court Justice Clarence Thomas wrote a lengthy opinion in *Box v. Planned Parenthood of Indiana and Kentucky* citing the eugenic roots of abortion to dispose of minorities, the poor, and the disabled.[31] The case handed down a two-part ruling on Indiana's abortion law, upholding dignity for fetal remains of abortions to be buried or cremated and unfortunately striking down the "nondiscrimination" provision of the law which prohibited abortions from being performed solely on the basis of sex, race, or disability. Thomas dedicated his opinion to demonstrate the slippery slope of doing away with the nondiscrimination provision: "This law and other laws like it promote a State's compelling interest in preventing abortion from becoming a tool of modern-day eugenics."

However, the eugenic efforts of abortion do not stop in our country. Such discrimination is happening all over the globe. The country of Iceland recently boasted that they had eradicated persons with Down syndrome due to early embryonic detection that led mothers to abort nearly 100 percent of the time.[32] In countries where there is a gender bias for males, particularly in East Asian countries, sex-selective abortions frequently occur if the baby is a girl. This has caused a disproportionate ratio of males to females in some of these countries, making it hard for men to find wives, and vice-versa. There are nearly 36 million more males than there are females in China due to China's previous "one-child policy."[33] Worldwide, there are an estimated 140 million missing girls due to sex-selective abortions.[34] (Research results vary and the number may be even higher. See note 13 in chapter 2.)

Sex-selective abortion practices also carry over into the United States as people from other countries immigrate here. The pro-life movement has championed discrimination laws that would prevent the termination of babies who are unwanted simply due to race, sex, or genetic anomalies that produce disabilities. Several states in the US have even passed their own versions of nondiscrimination abortion bills.[35] Sadly, litigation from Planned Parenthood and other abortion advocates committed to abortion on demand are currently preventing the bills' enaction.[36]

It is also a poorly kept secret that the United States and other developed countries that contribute to international agencies distributing aid to poverty- or conflict-ridden regions often do so with the strings of abortion and contraception attached. The Trump administration reversed many of the longstanding practices that allowed access to abortion services to be a prerequisite for receiving aid. In fact, this administration took the unprecedented step of rebuking the United Nations for equating abortion as "essential aid" next to food and water for countries in desperate need of basic resources, especially amid the coronavirus pandemic.[37] Under the Trump administration, America removed itself from the list of nations active in the global abortion agenda and would not fund international abortions.[38] But wealthy elites like Bill and Melinda Gates of the Gates Foundation continue to advocate for abortion efforts around the world couched in the vision of education and "quality healthcare."[39]

Continuing with the same Malthusian ideal, abortion is supported by progressives as a tool in curbing climate change. Yes, you heard that right: they wish to kill the people to save the environment. At a presidential town hall hosted by CNN, then-Democratic presidential hopeful Bernie Sanders was asked if curbing "population growth" was part of his "plan to address climate catastrophe." "The answer is yes," Sanders answered. He unashamedly endorsed abortion as part of his "plan to address climate catastrophe." His response, of course, continued with the guise of the right of women to control their own bodies. Sanders called efforts to restrict funds for overseas abortions as "absurd . . . especially in poor countries."[40] Former Vice President Al Gore wrote in his 1992 book, "No goal is more crucial to healing the global environment than stabilizing human population."[41] The Chinese Communist Party (CCP) was well ahead of Gore, implementing its infamous one-child policy on Chinese families that sadly led to forced abortions, sex-selective abortions, and forced sterilizations. Though this policy has since been changed,[42] its harmful effects cannot be undone. Under the CCP's vision for human dignity, one's value is not determined by intrinsic worth but by one's productivity. As former American Eugenics Society head and Population Council president Fredrick Osborn said, "Birth control and abortion are turning out to be great eugenic advances of our time."[43]

Conclusion

There is not enough room in this book to detail all the entanglements of support for abortion toward eugenic purposes under the guise of "women's reproductive health." Suffice it to say that abortion has become the primary tool to advance many evils in human hearts. It has given society consolation to worship the created (earth and self) instead of the Creator (God), who is the ruler and sustainer of all creation (Rom. 1:25; Col. 1:16–17). Jesus said that we will always have those who are poor among us (Mark 14:7). There is no cure for poverty except for the generosity of others (Lev. 19:10; 23:22), and people's value is not determined by the degree to which they are thought to burden society. Abortion sends the subliminal message that it is better for children to be dead than to live in poverty or to be unwanted.

Many have overcome obstacles, such as dire poverty. Moreover, it is a lie to say one's life does not matter. All lives matter to God, who creates everyone in His own image (Gen. 1:26). Abortion is one of

Satan's most effective tools as he works to "steal and kill and destroy" (John 10:10). Humanity, and society at large, will only flourish when we accept God's truth and commit to putting it into practice.

CLAIM 7

The Pro-Life Movement Doesn't Care about Social Justice

18

The Voices and Values of the New Pro-Life Generation

—Charlotte Pence Bond—

Young people search for more. It is not enough for a business to create a product that is a good idea, or that solves a problem, or that serves a need. It is not enough even for movies to be entertaining. For both millennials and "zoomers" of Generation Z, every industry and medium should provide a message, and that message should help disadvantaged people—specifically those considered to be victims of oppression—by providing them with equal opportunity for achievement and success.

Whether they are deciding where to shop, eat, work, or worship, many millennials (those who entered adulthood soon after the start of the new millennium) are more interested in an organization's overall commitment to doing good in the community than in anything else. According to a 2019 study by the Case Foundation, 90 percent of millennials are more motivated to give on the basis of a "compelling mission" than the identity of an organization.[1]

This attachment to a cause extends beyond the millennial generation and into Generation Z. Young people are becoming increasingly more interested in how their actions affect the well-being of others, both in America and across the globe. Thanks to investigative films and broader efforts to educate the public on the inhumane working conditions of sweatshops and foreign factories—some of which manufacture food, clothes, and everyday items sold in major department stores—high school and college students have begun to see that some of the companies they support take advantage of labor practices that are unsafe and immoral, and actually illegal in the United States. Instead of simply accepting or ignoring this reality, they have sought to lessen the negative impact consumerism has on others. They have even found ways to create change, whether by highlighting fair-trade businesses or by starting clubs on campuses where students discuss these problems and how to fix them.

Young Americans believe their actions matter, and that they can be the ones to effect change in the world. Not only do they understand this to be possible, but they view their wider role and responsibilities in society as things that need to be constantly considered. Their activism—their commitment to combating social injustices—defines who they are as people just as much as it defines the kind of world in which they want to live.

Abortion as Social Injustice

The term "social justice" is defined as "a state or doctrine of egalitarianism."[2] Accordingly, social justice movements seek to remedy social injustices by promoting equality in society. Abortion undermines a state of social justice because it is a practice that creates inequalities between people groups—both born and unborn. Accordingly, the pro-life movement is a social justice movement because it seeks to expose and overturn the practices of social injustice in order to provide fairness to all human beings. In fact, as we'll see below, the pro-life movement shares many of the same features that characterize other social justice movements in today's society.

1. Social justice movements seek to prevent human rights violations, and the same is true of the pro-life movement. The pro-choice coalition has done its best to dehumanize preborn children, and in doing so, it has become easier to bypass the social injustices involved in abortion. The focus of abortion defenders is normally on the rights of the woman who is making the difficult decision to end her pregnancy. They argue that a woman is in charge of her body, and therefore, it should be her choice to do with her body what she wants. Their concern also stems from the horrific experiences of those who had unsafe abortions when the procedure was illegal. Women seeking "back-alley" abortions often did so through the aid of underground organizations operating in unhygienic and dangerous conditions. Sadly, these women sometimes refused to seek medical help even if required, resulting in major health complications or death.[3]

The past horrors of back-alley abortions are a tragedy in the history of our nation and should not be forgotten. But this tragedy worsened when our nation legalized abortion, thus declaring that human rights do not begin in the womb, and that not all human life is equal. Abortion takes the human right to life away from a child, from someone who is too vulnerable to speak for himself or herself. Unborn children cannot advocate on behalf of their right to live. They cannot consent to what is being done to them. They do not have authority over their own bodies. They do not have agency or autonomy. The person in power over them decides what their future will hold without giving them a say in the matter. They are in a position of weakness where abuse can easily take place. Indeed, an aborted child is a *victim* in the same sense that millennials have learned to apply the term to other social justice issues.

Victimizing unborn children goes against our country's entire philosophy of freedom and liberty, and millennials are starting not only to notice this inconsistency, but to address it. The rising pro-life movement does not wish to minimize the terrible experiences of women who sought abortions in a world in which it was illegal. Rather, it puts the onus on this generation—on us—to stand up and not allow this injustice to further harm our society. Abortion, then, is clearly a violation of social justice, which makes the pro-life movement a social justice movement.

2. Social justice movements seek to address societal problems for which the symptoms are dealt with but the underlying cause remains uncured, and the same is true of the pro-life movement. Legalized, frequent abortion does not address the systemic problem that comes from the shame and burden of an unplanned pregnancy. A woman does not decide to go forward with an abortion for no reason. There are other cultural factors—such as popular-culture messaging that celebrates abortion and the promotion of chemical abortion on college campuses—that lead to this choice. But when abortion is readily available in surgical or chemical form, none of these other issues is addressed. Instead, abortion presents itself as a band-aid solution, attempting to cover up the problem for a moment, but it does not solve any of the larger cultural issues at play. In this way, abortion once again fits into the social justice narrative, making the pro-life movement a social justice movement.

3. *Social justice movements oppose organizations and structures that wield power in a way that harms people, and the same is true of the pro-life movement.* Planned Parenthood is a large corporation that receives taxpayer dollars in order to perform various health services, and most notably, abortions. However, in recent years, the public's use of Planned Parenthood for services other than abortion, like cancer screenings and prevention, has decreased significantly. In its 2011–2012 Annual Report, Planned Parenthood recorded that 12 percent of its services were for cancer screenings and prevention.[4] In its 2014–2015 report, this dropped to 7 percent,[5] then to 6.3 percent in 2017–2018.[6] Planned Parenthood's report for 2018–2019, showed that only 6 percent of its services were for cancer screenings and prevention.[7] In the same reports, abortion services climbed. As the Heritage Foundation reports, "Planned Parenthood affiliates performed 345,672 abortions from Oct. 1, 2017, to Sept. 30, 2018—the highest number of abortions ever reported in a single year"[8] (for any one organization). It is clear that this large organization is making abortion its financial focus. Planned Parenthood fits the role of a large organization that exploits vulnerable people while taking money from the general citizenry in the process.

Another way in which the abortion industry is seeking to reach young women is through the abortion pill. In 2017, 39 percent of all abortions were performed with the abortion pill.[9] Women are told that this is noninvasive and similar to a heavy period, but it isn't. It is often extremely painful, dangerous, and disturbing. I have spoken to women who have had chemical abortions, and healthcare employees who work with them, and the experience is often not the easy one that the abortion industry touts. I have been told[10] by pro-life workers, that a woman's home, bathroom, or dorm room becomes the area where an abortion takes place and she is essentially the abortionist. It is a lonely and heartbreaking experience, and women should be made more aware of the physical and emotional complications that can arise from chemical abortions.

This is not to say that everyone who works for Planned Parenthood is a bad person—far from it. Most men and women who work in the abortion industry truly believe that they are helping women escape a bad situation and improve their lives. I have spoken to people who have worked in the industry and have left when they decided they could no longer remain in such a hopeless work environment. These men and women are not to be judged, but it is important that we spread the facts about the alternatives to abortion and promote programs that help women with unplanned pregnancies, in order to show them that there are other options apart from abortion.

The reach of the pro-abortion culture has expanded outside of healthcare and has become a cultural topic. It is no longer something that has stayed in the medical world. Hollywood and pop culture have used their reach in a propagandist manner, with celebrities speaking about their personal experiences. This is another power structure—and it is used to spread misinformation that will ultimately harm women.

If the pro-choice movement has the cultural megaphone, young women will be naïvely pressured into a procedure that is more costly than they realize. The pro-life movement seeks to restrict the power of these proponents of social injustice, which makes the pro-life movement a social justice movement.

4. Social justice movements provide a voice for the voiceless, and the same is true of the pro-life movement. Abortion fails to give a voice to unborn children. That should be obvious, and should not be overlooked. But the "voiceless person" of abortion is not only the unborn child, it is also the woman who is not given the space to grieve the loss of her child, to understand what happened to her, and to come forward with her story. Abortion is trauma and it should be treated that way in our society. Sadly, it has come to be celebrated in a way that makes women with negative experiences and regrets feel as if they are the exception and have nowhere to go. This is another form of oppression—of silencing those that do not fit the overarching narrative of the powerful.

The Shout Your Abortion movement claims to help empower women to share their stories, but the movement's website contains many accounts that are heartbreaking to read.[11] The stories are moving, and people often anonymously submit their abortion experiences. Women who undergo an abortion are not the perpetrators in this social justice cause. They are not the people this movement should be fighting against. Rather, they are victims, and so are their unborn children. They are victims because they have been told a lie—that abortion is simple, easy, and the best option for their lives. Many women exit abortion clinics in overwhelming pain, and often they have no one to tell. The pro-life movement seeks to give voice to such social injustice, which makes the pro-life movement a social justice movement.

5. *Social justice movements are at their best when they remember the living, walking, breathing victims of tragedies and do all they can to help them recover, and the same is true of the pro-life movement.* When women and men are able to find healing from abortion, the trauma of this experience doesn't have to carry as much weight into their future lives. Their pain can be redeemed, and their stories can be used to help other men and women who find themselves in similarly heartbreaking situations. Various counseling centers, such as Project

Rachel,[12] provide post-abortive support for men and women, while Heartbeat International provides resources for people to find ways to heal from their heartache. The pro-life movement seeks to provide healing for victims of such social injustices, which makes the pro-life movement a social justice movement.

6. Social justice movements understand the legal reality in which they are fighting, and the same is true of the pro-life movement. In the 1990s, President Bill Clinton declared that abortion should be "safe, legal, and rare." We have seen this perspective almost disappear among Democrats in recent years, and it is important to take note of this shift and attempt to understand what it means for human rights.

Many on the liberal left have feared the reversal of the *Roe v. Wade* Supreme Court ruling for years. They have used propagandist tactics to scare women into believing that the world will become a dystopian-like reality if the Supreme Court decision were reversed. The reality is that overturning *Roe* would simply put the legislative decisions about abortion back in the hands of individual states.

In early 2020, Democrats in the Senate prevented the Born-Alive Abortion Survivors Protection Act from passing. The bill stated that doctors would be required to care for an infant who survives an abortion and treat the child as they would any other patient. A law such as this should be accepted by people on all sides of the abortion debate, but clearly our culture has become polarized to the point of even resisting this compromise.

Oppressive structures often operate in similar ways. They begin by asking for only a small amount of power but end up taking more and more as the culture leans in their direction. As abortion has become more mainstream and culturally acceptable, the pro-choice coalition has likewise sought greater and greater legislative progress. The pro-life movement is fully aware of the legal history of the social injustice it seeks to remedy, which makes the pro-life movement a social justice movement.

7. Social justice movements not only use culture and politics to change the narrative of the public mindset, they also use scientific advancements, and the same is true of the pro-life movement. Change that will make an impact must always be multifaceted, and millennials understand this better than anyone. They are constantly investigating organizations, as well as examining their own actions, to see how they are affecting disadvantaged communities. They understand that they are as much a player in promoting or preventing justice as are large corporations. Because of this, they are able to see the correlation between many different areas of life and how these avenues combine to create a cultural belief.

The main arguments for the pro-life movement used to be based on religious convictions. There is nothing wrong with this, for religious values are certainly a crucial part of the fight for human rights. However, making advancements in science as well as improving access to child care, adoption, and maternal healthcare can also significantly contribute to the reasons for people to choose life. Millennials understand this, though for them making abortion illegal is only the first step. It is also the mission of the new pro-life movement to make abortion, as Students for Life of America puts it, "unthinkable." In recent years, the narrative behind this has changed in a way that will help young men and women become pro-life.

The pro-choice movement began, in many ways, with the narrative that an unborn child is a collection of cells and tissue. I remember that when I was in elementary school, a young boy once told me that a baby wasn't alive before it was born. I assume he heard this from one of his parents or another adult in his life, but this was a commonly held belief only a few short years ago. That argument has been debunked by advancements in science—and common sense—but the sentiment remains in popular culture.

Abortion facilities and their websites often refer to "pregnancies" instead of "unborn children." When they describe the child, they use the term "fetus" only when entirely necessary. Using medical jargon like this, in place of humanizing language, creates a detached mindset for the abortionist. It also creates the kind of sterile environment that causes a woman to believe the decision to abort concerns only what is best for her health and life. Instead, the decision involves another human life and often results in heartache and unspoken pain.

Scientific advancements have improved our understanding of pregnancy, and ultrasounds have become even more vivid and realistic. Due to such technological progress, pro-lifers have insisted on laws that will give women a better understanding of their options, and a clearer picture of what abortion really is. This is how social justice movements effectively advance their cause, which makes the pro-life movement a social justice movement.

Young People Rising Up

When I was in college, I once saw a sticker in someone's apartment that I will always remember. It read, "I am the Pro-Life Generation." I am not sure where the person got it or if it was part of a protest or rally, but it was the first time I had seen those words so openly stated. I remember thinking, *Could we be?* Could we be the generation that not only saw an end to the legal practice of abortion, but stood up as a body, as a unit, to say that the injustices we are witnessing are not to be tolerated any longer?

It was the first time I realized that being pro-life could be *cool.* And that I wasn't alone. If it was a generational movement, if there were people my age who would proudly stand up and say that this is an injustice that needs to end, then maybe a difference really could be made.

Social justice movements find their footing because they are in fact a *movement,* a group, a body of people joining together with a rallying cry. When like-minded people discover one another—whether at a protest or a campus chapter or in a conversation—it is a powerful catalyst for change to occur. For millennials to attach to the issue of abortion, there must be people who are willing to be vocal about its eradication with them, so they are not alone.

Movements also need leaders. Social justice movements are often led by men and women—some quite young—who are able to reveal, often through covert action, that an injustice is taking place and are then able to convince others to join their cause. The pro-life generation has seen many such young men and women put themselves at the forefront and take charge on the difficult issue of abortion. With these young people calling attention to the negative effects of abortion on society and the inhumane practices of abortion clinics, millennials have heroes to emulate. They can learn how best to voice their arguments and answer the call to action.

Lila Rose is one of these leaders. She is the president of Live Action, a pro-life advocacy group she founded in 2003. She is best known for her undercover investigative reporting of abortion clinics in the United States. Rose, who posed as a sex abuse victim, filmed her conversations with clinic workers.[13] Later, she trained people to act as sex traffickers in order to reveal truths about the abortion industry. These videos were crucial in changing the narrative on anti-abortion activism. They allowed people to see that abortion clinics are not "for women" as much as their messaging might claim. Rose was a young woman who was fighting—and is still fighting—for young women by showing them the truth behind the claims of the abortion industry. Above all else, she is a fighter for social justice.

David Daleiden is another person who has used the power of undercover media to spread the truth about abortion. He even took his battle to the courts to fight Planned Parenthood. Daleiden's Center for Medical Progress released covert videos in which he filmed abortion industry workers admitting to trafficking fetal tissue. The act of selling human tissue is illegal and grossly immoral. The videos sparked outrage and led to investigations into Planned Parenthood clinics in various states.[14] Sadly, Daleiden was sued by the National Abortion Federation[15] and also faced criminal charges, including one felony charge, for his covert activism.[16]

Although Daleiden lost his court case in 2020, his efforts brought to light Planned Parenthood's business of selling fetal tissue for profit.

Students for Life of America (SFLA) is an organization that trains leaders in the pro-life movement. I have become more involved with this group in recent years and currently serve as a member of their National Advisory Board. I was initially connected to SFLA as an invited speaker and author, but when I became more familiar with the work they do, I wanted to become more involved. SFLA has chapters on college campuses all over the United States. They train students how to discuss pro-life issues and how to answer hard questions in conversation with friends and peers. This is extremely important, because young people will be challenged. But when equipped to speak about human rights, they will have the confidence to respond with intelligence, kindness, and clarity.

SFLA and their chapters also care about the future of the country. Their organization works hard to overturn the *Roe v. Wade* ruling, but they also recently published a "Blueprint for a Post-*Roe* America" that outlines how they can help women in vulnerable positions once *Roe v. Wade* is overturned.[17]

After the 1973 Supreme Court decision legalized abortion in all fifty states, the pro-life movement truly began. People began to voice their concerns about living in a country where abortion was legal. One of the major ways in which this was done was through protests and gatherings like the March for Life. The March for Life began in 1974, the year after *Roe v. Wade* was decided. I recently spoke to Reverend Frank Pavone, a priest and leader in the pro-life movement, about the impact of this campaign on his ministry. This is what he shared with me and he gave me permission to quote him:

> The event that galvanized my interest and participation in the pro-life movement, eventually leading me to commit my whole life and ministry to ending abortion, was the March for Life of 1976. It was the third annual March for Life in Washington DC, and the first thing I remember about it was that it was cold [outside]. But far warmer were the hearts of the participants: hearts that were at the same time broken but joyful. As St. Paul urged the Thessalonians, we grieve, but with hope. . . . It taught me what I've often repeated in my talks: we are not just working for victory; we are working from victory. Victory is our starting point, because Christ is risen and is with us, and death has been conquered. And as we battle the evil of abortion, we already have an anticipatory joy of the final victory of good and of life.

Since the beginning of the pro-life movement, the March for Life has grown dramatically—and young people from schools and youth groups all around America make the trek every year to brave the Washington, DC winter as they protest at the nation's capital for the right of all human beings to live freely. The March for Life rarely gets the attention it deserves. In recent years, prominent politicians have attended the event, but nonetheless, the mainstream media continues to ignore the large numbers of people who gather.

This is another characteristic of a social justice campaign—the loudest and most powerful parts of society largely ignore the people's outcries. Although there are many outlets that report on the march, there is typically much more attention paid to liberal causes. This should not surprise anyone who has followed campaigns for justice throughout history. When there is an overarching cultural narrative that is more accepted by the elite—whether these elites are in Hollywood, the nation's capital, or other large institutions—the voices of those who are fighting for something that is less popular are often drowned out. The options, then, remain clear: the protestors can give up or they can try harder—and play smarter. The latter is exactly what the pro-life movement has done in recent years, that is, expanding its reach into the younger generation and doing so in a way that appeals to them on a human level rather than only from a legislative distance.

Last year, I spoke to groups of students who attended the March for Life. As I spoke, I saw faces staring intently up at me, surrounded by their friends and fellow pro-lifers. But what stuck out to me most was how intensely they appeared to pay attention to what I was saying—not because of who I am or because of the choice of my words alone, but because I did my best to acknowledge their struggles and to remind them that they are not alone. Those students and young people were returning to their own states, schools, and workplaces the next day. They were going back into a culture that not only rejects their message, but actively challenges it and claims that they lack empathy and kindness because of it.

As I looked out across that room of young people, I was humbled. They are much braver than I was at their age. I attended the March for Life during my youth, and though at the time I was in agreement with the pro-life position, I wasn't as vocal or involved as they are now. In the hallways of my high school and on my college campus, I was afraid to voice my beliefs about abortion. I, like so many Americans, feared that I would be viewed as judgmental.

While I tried my best to encourage the students that day, I couldn't help but think how much they were going to need it. The world is pushing back against them harder than ever before, but, as with every fight for human rights, the necessary response is to push right back and to do so in a way that affects real, lasting change. Organizations that gather millennials together in the way that the March for Life does are putting in the hard work that will endure into the future. These people are changing the culture right where it is formed—in the minds of young people. But they aren't only going to large gatherings, they are going to campuses and homes and taking the pro-life message with them.

Conclusion

The legalization of abortion not only resulted in a devastating loss of life in our country, but it created a nation whose culture celebrates injustice in the name of women's rights. This has had an impact on young women, where no longer is the "safe, legal, rare" argument even considered. Abortion is seen not only to be necessary, but good.

And this is where the current social justice fight truly lies. There are advances that need to occur in order to change our country's laws on human rights for the unborn, but a cultural shift is more urgent and more important—and it will only be successful if it targets the younger generation.

Young people are beginning to see that a culture of abortion is a culture of social injustice. It leads to inequality for disadvantaged groups, it victimizes those who are vulnerable, and it takes away autonomy and agency from those who can't defend themselves. It also provides a defeatist narrative—one that says someone cannot rise to the unforeseen challenges and trials that life brings.

Social justice causes are formed in order to eradicate oppressive forces—whether they are systemic, institutional, or historical. Abortion is oppression. Thankfully, young people are increasingly rising up against a culture of inequality. They are noticing the ways in which abortion not only ends a life, but deteriorates communities, hurts women, and harms families.

Fighting for justice is empowering, and abortion is a great hindrance to empowerment. When young people become involved in this movement, they join the ranks of those fighting for what will be remembered as the social justice issue of our time.

19

The Hands and Feet of Jesus: How Pregnancy Centers Care for Women and Men

—Sandy Christiansen—

"Two lines, that means I'm pregnant! This can't be happening!" Nina immediately began googling in search of help. She saw an ad that read, "Pregnant and unsure what to do? We can help." She dialed the number and scheduled a same-day appointment. As Nina sat in the waiting room of the pregnancy center, she read an online review about it. "All they care about is your baby. They will do everything they can to keep you from getting an abortion." Nina panicked and was getting up to leave when the client advocate approached her.[1] The client advocate listened to her concerns and reassured Nina that she could leave at any time and that under no circumstances would she be subjected to coercion or other forms of pressure. Nina decided not to leave. At the end of her visit, she exclaimed, "I'm so glad I stayed! That review was completely wrong. I felt safe here and know that you truly care about my well-being, and not just about my baby's life."

The pro-life movement has faced opposition since its inception. The societal upheaval of the 1960s laid the groundwork for the passage of *Roe v. Wade*, which elevated a woman's personal privacy over the life of her unborn child. The battle lines were drawn and the persistent mantra began: *the pro-life movement doesn't care about women, only about the baby*. Abortion advocates maintained: *Where was the love and compassion for the single mother living on welfare? Does the pro-life community care about women trapped in violent relationships? Women deserve choice. Abortion is a safe option for women, so why the lies about associated risks?* The reality is that the pro-life movement does care about the men and women who are convinced that abortion is their best choice. And one of the obvious proofs for this concern is the work of pregnancy centers.

Pregnancy centers are on the front lines of the pro-life movement, providing compassion, hope, and help to women and men considering abortion. There are over 2,700 pregnancy centers in North America, and over 1,100 are affiliates of Care Net—the largest evangelical network of pregnancy centers in the United States, for which I serve as National Medical Director. The National Institutes of Family Life Advocates (NIFLA) and Heartbeat International, along with Care Net, comprise the three largest networks of affiliate organizations for pregnancy centers and provide best practice guidelines and training to equip centers with excellence.

But despite their faithful service within communities, pregnancy centers continue to be a target of criticism and legislative attacks. Critics claim that the pro-life community and pregnancy centers "only care about the baby" and aren't concerned about the broader issues that affect the lives of the women and men who enter their facilities. Detractors propagate misinformation, like that conveyed in the misleading online review that Nina read. A closer look at the work of pregnancy centers reveals a dramatically different reality.

Pregnancy centers understand the complexities of their clients' lives and how health concerns, traumas, social determinants, and other factors interplay to create barriers to health and thriving. Pregnancy centers seek to address the chaos and struggles clients face and to help them craft solutions that promote health and well-being, build resilience, strengthen relationships, and foster healthy families. Every day, pregnancy centers open their doors ready to serve their clients and invest time and energy actively addressing many of the commonly recognized inequalities that drive the pursuit of social justice.[2] The 2,700 community-based pregnancy centers accomplish this through the direct delivery of free medical services, the provision of coaching and recovery programs, the administration of educational programs, the furnishing of material support, and by making referrals for ongoing care within the community.

The Mission of Pregnancy Centers & Social Justice

Tim Keller wrote, "If you are trying to live a life in accordance with the Bible, the concept and call to justice are inescapable. We do justice when we give all human beings their due as creations of God. Doing justice includes not only the righting of wrongs but generosity and social concern, especially toward the poor and vulnerable."[3]

Annually, over 860,000 abortions occur in the US alone.[4] There are no more vulnerable humans in the world than the unborn. How should Christians respond to this injustice? How might they show generosity and social concern for these creations of God? What about the men and women who are hurt physically, emotionally, and spiritually by abortion? What does justice look like for them? While there are many appropriate responses and solutions, pregnancy centers model their approach after the ministry of Jesus.

Christians understand that apart from the gospel of Jesus Christ, there is no justice. As Jesus spread the gospel message, His heart was moved with compassion for hurting people. He showed us how to love and gave us a great example in the Good Samaritan (Luke 10:30–37). Filled with compassion and fueled by love of Jesus Christ, pregnancy centers—much like the Good Samaritan—provide physical, emotional, and spiritual support to help people live their best lives and experience what John 10:10 describes as living "abundantly."

Three words characterize pregnancy center work: *compassion, hope*, and *help*. Unencumbered by politics or other socioeconomic barriers, pregnancy centers provide the person-to-person connection of the pro-life movement. Centers engage clients with Christ-inspired compassion and respect their dignity and worth as people made in the image of God. The hearts of pregnancy center workers break for the women and men who believe that abortion is the answer to their perceived problem and for the unborn child who may never be given a chance at life. They know that both the mom and the baby are in need of rescue, and this starts with the woman who is in an abusive relationship, who is already caring for one or more child, and who sees abortion as her only solution. She needs a safe place to address her physical, emotional, and spiritual health and to get all the facts as she thinks through this critical decision. At the center, clients find a judgment-free zone and enter a sanctuary where they can slow down and sort things out.

Contrary to critics who maintain that pregnancy centers only care about the woman until she says she'll carry her baby rather than abort, centers invest time and money into providing ongoing support to help their clients thrive. This support takes many forms: medical services, mental health screenings, pregnancy decision coaching, post-abortive counseling, educational classes, baby clothes and material support, referrals for further medical care, and more.

Medical Services

Pregnancy center medical clinics provide an important public service for women who are considering abortion and for those who fall through the cracks in the healthcare system, lacking ready access to pregnancy support and prenatal care. They address healthcare disparities of the disenfranchised and marginalized within their communities, who comprise a majority of their clients. The medical services are provided under the license and authority of a physician and adhere to all applicable laws.

The very first pregnancy centers provided free pregnancy tests for their clients. Today, nearly 80 percent of centers perform ultrasound exams to confirm pregnancy. In 2019, medical pregnancy clinics provided 486,000 free ultrasound examinations with an estimated cost value of $121 million.[5] The introduction of ultrasound exams has been a game-changer for parents considering abortion. When an expectant parent sees their baby's heart beating during an ultrasound exam, any doubt about this being "just a blob of tissue" disappears. This knowledge is powerful and indisputable.

Sexually transmitted infections have reached epidemic proportions in the United States.[6] One-third of centers provide testing for common sexually transmitted diseases and are often the only free option where people may receive confidential testing.[7] Clients receive factual information about healthy sexuality and the risks associated with their lifestyle choices. Lifestyle coaching and education are provided for clients who desire to make changes. Following a trend to offer faith-based alternative healthcare options to communities, some centers have expanded their medical services to include well-woman exams, prenatal care, and pap testing.[8]

Many clients who come to pregnancy centers for care do not have health insurance and cannot afford to pay out of pocket to see a physician. Pregnancy centers are committed to removing financial barriers by providing services at no charge to clients. In 2019, pregnancy centers provided over $266,000,000 worth of services and material support to clients![9] This included over 730,000 pregnancy tests, 486,000 ultrasound exams, and 160,000 sexually transmitted disease tests.[10]

Each of these numbers represents real people with real stories and, in many cases, lives saved. Take, for example, the story of Carrie, who was working at a fast-food restaurant to help support her two children when she missed her period. After taking a pregnancy test, she smiled ruefully; the timing wasn't good, but she saw children as a gift from God. When Carrie told her husband about being pregnant, he was uncertain how they could have another child at this time. Feeling stressed, she came to the center for a pregnancy test and ultrasound exam to confirm her pregnancy. As I met with Carrie, I shared information about abortion procedures, risks, and alternatives. During her ultrasound exam, she smiled when she saw her baby. In her heart, she was determined to trust God to provide. Her husband's initial reluctance to have another child was subsequently replaced by the joy of a new addition to the family.

Carrie received critical medical services that helped her have a healthy pregnancy. Early entry into prenatal care positively correlates with improved medical outcomes.[11] She received a free pregnancy test, a clinical evaluation, blood pressure assessment, an ultrasound exam to confirm pregnancy, prenatal vitamins, and was referred for prenatal care. Carrie also received the emotional and spiritual support she needed to remain steadfast in her personal convictions to choose life for her baby.

In 2019, pregnancy centers administered over 700,000 free pregnancy tests with an estimated visit value of over $6.5 million.[12] Each of these was provided free of charge to the client. This is because pregnancy centers are not about transactional relationships with clients. Instead, they seek to introduce clients to the One who can transform their lives and circumstances. Unlike Planned Parenthood's service model, which is essentially "come as you are, don't change, come back again," Care Net's approach can be summed as, "come as you are, encounter Christ, and be transformed to live the abundant life."

Screening for Critical Public Health Issues

Like many people, pregnancy center clients lead complex and, at times, chaotic lives. Pregnancy centers provide important public health services to the community by screening clients for mental health issues, substance abuse, sexual assault, intimate partner violence, and human trafficking. Center workers are trained to approach people holistically, attending to their physical, emotional, and spiritual needs and addressing social determinants to their health and welfare. Client advocates learn how to identify those who require immediate intervention or referrals for appropriate follow-up care, including legal reporting.

The path that leads to a pregnancy at the age of sixteen is often full of twists and turns and cannot be unraveled by a one-dimensional solution. Depression and suicide rates are high among today's youth, as are substance abuse issues, and a pregnancy scare may exacerbate these problems. During the pregnancy test visit, clients are often screened for common issues which could remain undetected and lead to serious consequences.

Women experiencing lack of support or pressure to abort from their partners are more likely to choose abortion.[13] Women who face intimate partner violence are significantly more likely to choose abortion.[14] Having prior mental health challenges is also one risk factor for experiencing mental health challenges after abortion. These issues clearly play a role in the woman's abortion decision and thus are critical to identify and address. Many centers provide training in trauma-informed coaching to equip client advocates to identify and address the specific adverse situations a client is experiencing. Intentionally asking clients about these and other serious issues can break the cycle of silence and fear. Centers help clients connect with the long-term support they need to address the problem and begin their journey toward health and safety. Clients are referred to safe houses, legal support, medical care, mental health support, and other resources for effecting change in their lives.

Coerced or forced abortion is a problem, particularly for minors and those caught up in sex trafficking.[15] Minors are often unaware that no one may force them to have an abortion.[16] Pregnancy centers are positioned to educate and empower their clients in making a decision they can live with long term. All these services provide important solutions for healthcare disparities that are common among the clients of pregnancy centers.

Pregnancy Decision Support and Options Coaching

At a pregnancy center, clients learn the truth about abortion procedures and are educated about how an abortion can affect their long-term health. Many women are unaware that by choosing abortion they will have an increased risk of preterm birth with a subsequent pregnancy, of future development of breast cancer, and of depression, anxiety, substance abuse, and suicidal thoughts and behaviors.[17] Too often, center workers hear the stories of women who say, "If I had only known this, I wouldn't have had the abortion." As a physician dedicated to women's health, I am committed to defend and uphold a woman's right to be given full information about how a medication or procedure may impact her body and overall health.

For the woman who is considering abortion, the pregnancy center is a safe place to hear about her options. Unlike abortion clinics that stand to gain financially by an abortion decision, pregnancy center clients receive free services and have the opportunity to hear the facts about their options: parenting, adoption, and abortion.[18] Pregnancy centers are dedicated to equipping men and women with all the facts about abortion and fetal development so they can make an informed decision.[19]

Pathways to Abortion Recovery and Healing

One of the most beautiful aspects of pregnancy center work is that of abortion recovery. Women who have experienced abortion, together with their partners or family members who participated in the abortion decision, may struggle with the choice they made. After abortion, some say they initially felt relief and looked forward to their lives returning to normal. But other women report negative emotions after abortion that linger unresolved. For some, problems related to their abortion emerge months or even years later.[20]

While many abortion recovery resources exist, Care Net's book *Forgiven and Set Free,* authored by Linda Cochrane, is the most popular, according to a survey of US pregnancy centers. Through spiritually focused recovery, thousands of women and men have experienced freedom from the shame and guilt often associated with abortion.[21]

I have seen how women wrestle when considering abortion; it is not an easy decision for many. Diane's story says it all:

> When I found myself pregnant at sixteen years old, I was scared and needed a fast solution. I could not imagine having a child at my age, so I chose abortion. No one prepared me for what would happen or what I might feel during and after the procedure. I was shocked at the physical pain, but the emotional pain during and after the procedure was life changing.
>
> Fast forward twenty years. My husband and I began attending a local, nondenominational church and I found out that this church was very invested in a local pregnancy center. I signed up for the volunteer training. I'll never forget that the woman who called me about the training asked me if I had abortion in my past. I was totally taken aback. I said yes, expecting her to tell me that I couldn't be a part of this center; however, she asked me how I felt about my abortion and was I okay? I was speechless. No one had ever asked me how I felt about my abortion. I realized that I needed healing. Going through the post-abortion Bible study, God softened my heart, opened my eyes, and I learned who He truly was for the first time. I am now a pro-life Christian who has a heart for women (and men) facing unplanned pregnancies who need post-abortion healing, as well as the women who are so fiercely pro-choice and the abortion workers themselves. Praise God for His truth, mercy, grace and unconditional love!

Diane's story underscores the vital role of a relationship with Jesus Christ in transforming the hearts and minds of individuals either faced with a difficult pregnancy decision or reeling from the consequences of having made that decision. The gospel is integral to Care Net's mission.[22]

Care for Men

Men have strong ideas and feelings about fatherhood. Societal trends and mores that separate intimate sexual relations from relationship and commitment have done a disservice to men and women alike. Data support that women, men, and children thrive within the protective framework of a loving committed marriage relationship.[23] Care Net recognizes the critical role that men have when couples face a difficult pregnancy decision and encourage men to have a voice, take responsibility for their actions, and be a genuine support. Many of the reasons that women share for choosing abortion connect directly, or indirectly, to lack of partner support.[24]

Data are emerging that indicate men, too, can struggle after an abortion decision.[25] Laws and societal pressures have conditioned men to believe that the only thing they should say when their partner says she's pregnant is, "I'll support whatever decision you make." Guy Condon and David Hazard write in *Fatherhood Aborted*:

> When a man has fathered a child and that child's life is terminated by the unnatural and violent act of abortion, a destructive chain reaction silently begins in his life. . . . First, there is a deafening silence in our culture about the terrible aftershocks of abortion itself. . . . The sad truth is that many churches and individual Christians help keep this cultural silence in place. They're uncomfortable talking about abortion, sometimes

because they don't want to offend anyone or because they think it's better to keep their children from hearing about the harsh realities of life.[26]

Care Net has led the way in educating and equipping centers about the importance of the father's involvement in his partner's unplanned pregnancy. In our national survey of women who had abortions, it was shown that the father of the child was the most influential person in the mother's decision to abort. Nearly 70 percent of Care Net–affiliated centers have some type of outreach to men and fathers. These services may include individual options coaching and dad support classes. Care Net has developed educational pamphlets, videos, and other materials specifically designed to equip men to be supportive partners and excellent dads. Partners are often included in the ultrasound visit—this provides concrete evidence that he is indeed a father. Care Net data shows that women are significantly more likely to choose life when the father of the baby is included in their ultrasound appointment.

Education and Material Support

Like the Good Samaritan, pregnancy centers provide practical support for parents in need that extends well beyond the birth of a client's baby. In 2019, pregnancy centers provided parenting classes for over 1.7 million clients at an estimated cost of $51 million.[27] These classes help equip parents and build strong families. First-time single moms and young couples are particularly in need of mentors to guide them through their pregnancies and to help prepare them to care for an infant. Classes cover a wide range of topics, including pregnancy and birth, the first year of life, parenting, life skills, being a father and more. Expectant parents can learn about body changes in the first trimester of pregnancy, labor and delivery, how to bathe their baby, and milestones in childhood development. Class participants gain very practical knowledge that isn't readily available elsewhere, such as creating a budget, how to deal with childhood anger, single parenting during deployment, and more. For women and men who see their pregnancy as a crisis, preparing to take care of an infant can be overwhelming. Class facilitators provide important emotional support and encouragement giving clients an anchor during a time of flux and change. Participants not only gain important knowledge; they also develop a support network among fellow class participants and the facilitator. This practical support has helped thousands of clients take positive steps to improving their lives and building healthier families.

Providing material support for parents, infants, and children has been a mainstay of pregnancy centers. A short list of free support clients received in one year includes: 1.3 million packs of diapers, two million baby outfits, and 19,000 strollers.[28] The 2020 Charlotte Lozier Report notes that pregnancy centers provided 30,000 car seats to clients representing over $2.4 million![29] This just scratches the surface of the abundance that pregnancy centers shower on their clients each day. Visiting a center's baby boutique reveals hand-crocheted blankets, baby bouncers, pack and plays, cribs, baby shampoo, formula, diaper cream, maternity clothes, and lovingly arranged layettes for newborns, all of which are given away free of charge.

Pregnancy centers also partner with organizations that sometimes provide additional financial support for individuals and families. On top of receiving great medical care from the local Care Net center, Carrie (introduced above) was also blessed by the generosity of one of these partner institutions. During her exam, I asked Carrie about her future hopes and dreams. She shared that she was attending community college with the hopes of becoming an engineer one day. I told her about a special program that Regent University had developed with Care Net to provide scholarships for pregnancy center clients. She was very interested. We quickly pulled together all the requirements and submitted her application. Some weeks passed. Carrie entered prenatal care, enrolled in our center's Earn While You Learn pregnancy and parenting preparatory classes, and shopped at our baby boutique. I got a phone call that brought tears to my eyes: Carrie had been selected by Care Net to receive a Regent University four-year scholarship! When we told Carrie the news, she could not speak as the tears flowed. Carrie's future was secure, and she would realize her dream of completing her college education and becoming an engineer. Her story exemplifies the multi-pronged approach that typifies client care at a pregnancy center.

Connections with Community Resources

Sophia came to the center when she found out that she was pregnant. She didn't want to get an abortion, but thought she needed one because she couldn't see a way forward. "How can I raise a baby when I'm living in my car?" Pregnancy centers are ready to help women like Sophia. They are well connected within their communities, know the available resources, and are ready to advocate for the needs of their clients. In Sophia's case, several housing solutions emerged: a local nonprofit had a spot for her in their women's shelter, and a center volunteer knew of a friend from church who was ready to take her into her home as well. Once Sophia learned about these options and experienced the compassionate care at the pregnancy center, she was able to plan for her pregnancy.

Pregnancy centers across North America have developed extensive referral lists. These "care connections" can become the support network a client needs to believe that choosing life is realistic. Clients may receive a wide variety of support, including healthcare, prenatal care, assistance with procuring health insurance, mental health treatment, addiction recovery, intimate partner violence support, legal care, escape from trafficking, and more. Centers care deeply about all the needs of their clients and are ready to advocate for services within their communities.

While pregnancy centers are able to provide support for parents from the diagnosis of pregnancy through the first few years of the child's life, they aren't designed to provide long-term care for their clients. That is the work of the church. Care Net has developed a training program for churches called Making Life Disciples. This program equips church members to come alongside a person who is in a crisis pregnancy and provide long-term practical, spiritual, and emotional support, and ongoing discipleship.

Anne came to the Center for a pregnancy test and an ultrasound to confirm her pregnancy. Her face showed her stress and anguish as she told me her story. A mother of six children, including two sets of twins, Anne was working a full-time job at home while raising her children, conducting their schooling, and running the household. She received no material support from the children's father, who rarely even came around to visit. The COVID pandemic added to her stress.

She could not see how she could possibly raise one more child on her own. Although her boyfriend wanted her to carry, he was reluctant to provide much practical support. Feeling conflicted, she made an appointment for an abortion.

By God's grace, she came to us for an ultrasound before she went to the abortion clinic. During her ultrasound appointment, I shared with Anne the potential long-term risks associated with abortion. She was particularly at risk for emotional and psychological consequences because she was so conflicted about her decision and it was contrary to her values. She was moved by seeing the baby's beating heart.

After the ultrasound exam, she had shifted from abortion-minded to undecided about her pregnancy. We told Anne about Making Life Disciples, and she was interested. At the end of her visit, she allowed us to pray for her.

She then connected with a trained church volunteer who became the hands and feet of Jesus to her. The church volunteers made meals, did housework and yard work, carried trash to the dump, helped find child care, and supported her emotionally and spiritually. Anne did not keep the appointment for the abortion and, instead, decided to carry her baby and entered prenatal care.

During routine prenatal care testing, the doctors discovered that Anne's baby had severe problems and carried a life-limiting diagnosis. Once again, Anne was at a crossroads. Would she continue to carry a baby who was not expected to survive outside the womb?

Anne made the courageous decision to carry her baby, knowing that his life would likely be very short. The center provided perinatal hospice support throughout her pregnancy, helped her make a birth plan, and even helped her to plan to create special remembrances like molded hand and footprints at the time of birth.

During every step of this journey, Anne sought to trust God and exercise faith, even when she could not see how things could possibly work out. She is an inspiration to us. Her son only lived briefly after birth before passing into the arms of Jesus. She told us that she would not have been able to walk this path apart from her faith in God and without the help of the church and the pregnancy center.

Conclusion

Where can people in communities receive free medical services with no sliding scale? The 2020 Charlotte Lozier Institute impact report on 2,700 pregnancy centers across the United States tells an astounding story of unbridled compassion for people who need help and support with unexpected pregnancies, the lingering heartache of abortion, and building healthy families.

While the sheer numbers are impressive (nearly one million new clients served for an estimated value of over $28 million), the deeper value is harder to quantify.[30] Exit surveys give a glimpse of some of the intangibles that make all the difference between an ordinary physician's office or social service agency and the client experience at pregnancy centers:

> "I came into your office to confirm a pregnancy and get an ultrasound. I absolutely loved the care and attention and information I was given by all the staff at your office. I recently got a call from your office to see how I was doing and how my pregnancy was going, and it is going amazingly. I wanted to take the time to thank you and your staff for being such a caring team and very helpful, especially for someone who was new to the area and had nowhere to turn."

> "The receptionist and the client advocate were very respectful and kind. The doctor/nurse was very helpful because they helped explain my unanswered questions. They told me things in a way so I can understand and comprehend. I give my experience five stars! They care a lot about the people who walk through their doors."

> "The client advocate made me feel very comfortable. The doctor explained for me everything she was seeing in ultrasound. She was very clear and had a lot of patience. I received great quality services. I love that we prayed after my appointment."

The pro-life movement seeks to honor God by championing that which He holds dear: the sanctity of human life. There are many facets to this work—from those who are called to fight the battle in legislative halls and courts to those who steadfastly pray in silence before abortion clinics. Each facet is needed to add brilliance to the gem so that its beauty and light may be seen from all angles and vantage points. In the midst of the endless political rancor and societal division over abortion, pregnancy centers remain the calm in the eye of the storm.

Each day, these small nonprofit organizations faithfully serve women, men, and families providing compassion, hope, and help to all who enter their doors. Before a client ever comes to the center, she has been prayed over, prepared for, and loved. Inspired by Christ and empowered by the Holy Spirit, pregnancy center workers embody kindness, treating everyone with respect and dignity as image bearers of God. Centers address the needs of their clients by offering practical help and support. Medical services—such as pregnancy tests, ultrasound exams, infection testing, and screening for common issues such as mental health concerns—fulfill important client healthcare needs and promote well-being. Clients who choose to carry their pregnancies are offered classes to help equip them to raise a child. Helping clients overcome financial limitations, centers support families with baby supplies and equipment. Astoundingly, all these goods and services are delivered at no charge to the clients!

Across North America, pregnancy centers have no equal. Each of these nonprofit agencies (2,700 strong!) are united in a common purpose and together form a resilient force for good. Pregnancy centers help build strong communities one person at a time.

20

The Pro-Life Movement: A Last Line of Protection for Black Women and Their Babies

—Catherine Davis—

Despite what some people may believe, the pro-life movement is not a monolithic consortium made up of individuals and organizations who all walk in lockstep, ideologically aligned in every way. Pro-lifers, while against abortion, come from a variety of backgrounds, both secular and religious, and hold various viewpoints on any given issue.

But there is one thing many pro-lifers agree on—that the Black community has been and is being targeted by the abortion industry, and Planned Parenthood is leading the charge. Planned Parenthood has grown their business into being the largest provider of abortion in America, and as such they lead in messaging the reproductive rights (or justice) agenda. Another point on which most pro-lifers agree is that this targeting is achieving the goals intended, as more than twenty million Black lives have been taken at the hands of abortionists since *Roe v. Wade* was decided.

Recognizing that this targeting is happening *is* very different from understanding *how* it is happening right before our eyes. Planned Parenthood has taken care to disguise their service delivery in civil rights terminology. This was designed to assuage concerns some may have about the targeting. They have become masters at camouflaging abortion's deadly results by twisting the very arguments pro-lifers make and by shifting attention onto other social justice concerns. For example, they have accused pro-lifers of not caring about the children once they are born and have challenged pro-lifers on whether they have adopted children out of foster care. They have claimed that pro-lifers are really only pro-birth, for they leave poor children to fend for themselves, rather than providing resources to help them out of poverty. But these attempts to deflect cannot erase the fact that Planned Parenthood from its inception has been preying on Black women and their babies, for whom the pro-life movement is the last line of protection.

The Birth of the Negro Project

The targeting of Blacks by the American Birth Control League (later renamed Planned Parenthood) began in 1921, when the organization was founded by Margaret Sanger "to promote eugenic birth selection throughout the United States so that there may be more well born and fewer ill born children—a stronger, healthier and more intelligent race."[1] In 1939, they identified the target of their eugenic birth selection by launching the Negro Project, directing their messaging, finances, and facilities toward primarily Black women and babies.

The premise of the Negro Project was and is to hire ministers, doctors, and others of influence to "straighten it out" if it occurred to any of the more rebellious members of the community that the Birth Control League wanted to exterminate Blacks.[2] In the early days, they cited certain influential Black voices as advocates of birth control who could be trusted to "straighten out" any misperceptions of the league. In 1942, the name of the Birth Control League was changed to Planned Parenthood to disguise their eugenic roots after Adolph Hitler's determination to exterminate Jews, Blacks, the disabled, and others was exposed. Today, besides enlisting the aid of doctors and ministers, Planned Parenthood has expanded the Negro Project to include candidates for office and elected officials "who promise to go above and beyond to protect and expand health care access."[3]

For more than eighty years various members of the Black community have spoken against the Negro Project. Men and women of influence sounded the alarm, warning the Black community of a genocidal intent many believed was behind birth control and, later, abortion. Prominent men like Marcus Garvey, a well-known activist, vehemently opposed birth control. In 1932, Garvey was among the first Black leaders to make it known that Blacks could achieve political power in America through increasing their numbers in the population, not through birth control.

In a 1945 edition of the *Negro Digest*, Dr. Julian Lewis, the first Black professor at the University of Chicago, spoke against birth control, instead celebrating a "biologic victory for the Black man." The victory, he said, "tells how a race, acclimated for ages to one country, is able within a period of about 300 years to successfully establish itself in a wholly different land, a performance rarely, if ever, duplicated." He recognized "the precocious fertility of Negroes was exploited to its fullest capacity by avaricious slaveholders. It is said that the highest reproductivity ever observed was attained by slaves." That biologic victory resulted in the tripling of the Black population from 4,441,830 in 1860 to 12,865,518 in 1940. Lewis warned that "if an altered birthrate was maintained from year to year, Blacks would become an inconspicuous group in this nation. For these reasons Negroes must look askance at any proposals that threaten to reduce their birthrate."[4]

Dr. Charles Greenlee, William Bouie Haden, Erma Clardy Craven, Kay James, and Mildred Fay Jefferson were among a growing list of Blacks who joined the fight against birth control and abortion. As the threat grew, Ms. Craven warned that the "unborn Black baby is the real object of many abortionists. . . . Now, the womb of the poor black woman is seen as the latest battle ground for oppression."[5]

The Survival and Rebranding of the Negro Project

Exposing the eugenic impact of abortions on the Black community was not well received by those performing them. Over time, the abortion industry began expending resources to redirect the American culture toward acceptance of abortion as a norm that empowers women, especially Black women. This effort has increased considerably in recent years, and in direct response to the strategies of the pro-life movement.

For example, the abortion industry was caught off-guard in 2010 when eighty billboards were placed in Black neighborhoods across Atlanta that read, "Black Children Are an Endangered Species."[6] Those billboards were the most news-generating offering by pro-lifers that year. Print, television, and radio media covered the campaign, and abortion defenders struggled to respond to the facts presented. One response was the formation of the Trust Black Women partnership, a project of SisterSong, an organization heavily funded by Planned Parenthood and other abortion centered foundations.[7] The work of Trust Black Women resulted in the silencing of the billboard campaign and the defeat of subsequent legislative proposals to restrict abortion in Georgia.

Efforts to restyle the abortion industry have also been led by Loretta Ross, the former National Coordinator for SisterSong and the mother of the reproductive justice movement. Ross was the first abortion defender to deliberately craft messaging to reframe and rebrand Planned Parenthood's eugenic roots in terms of "reproductive health and justice." This messaging was then made the core argument against the message of abortion's genocidal impact on Black women and in support of abortion.[8]

In 2012, Cecile Richards, former president of Planned Parenthood, persuaded the Ford Foundation, on whose board she sits, to commission Belden Russonello Strategists to craft a more universal response. Introduced at a forum hosted by the women of the Congressional Black Caucus, the strategists rolled out language their foot soldiers could use that is still being recited today, such as "every community should have access to quality healthcare; cite historical disparities whenever the prolife community refers to the number of abortions on Black women; and challenge the other side to defend why they are contributing to making the disparities worse."[9] Rather than address their targeting of the Black community head-on, defenders of abortion began changing the conversation to issues that had little or no relevance to the question of abortion's impact on Black women and babies.

At the same time that they launched the attack against the billboards, Planned Parenthood activated a network in the mainstream media to suppress the voices of pro-life Black leaders. While almost every media outlet in the nation had reported the story about the "Black Children Are an Endangered Species" billboards, after the roll out of the Belden Russonello strategy very few, if any, national media carried stories on campaigns hosted by members of the National Black Pro-life Coalition, despite sending reporters to cover the events. A recent example included the 2019 National Day of Mourning. As commented in an opinion piece in the *Wall Street Journal*:

> Black pro-lifers, alas, are treated as if they don't exist. Quick example: How many outlets even reported the National Day of Mourning that concluded this past Saturday with a prayer service in Birmingham, Ala., for all the black lives lost to abortion? One of its leaders was Alveda King, a niece of Martin Luther King. Another was Catherine Davis of the Restoration Project, who notes that the estimated 20 million black abortions since *Roe v. Wade* in 1973 are more than the entire African-American population in 1960.[10]

The media reach of the abortion industry includes billboard companies that also began to suppress the pro-life messages that were so successful in the past. In 2017, Preterm (a Cleveland-based abortion facility) placed sixteen billboards in Black neighborhoods, declaring abortion sacred and a blessing, among other things.[11] In 2018, billboard advertising companies Outfront and Clear Channel refused to allow the pro-life Radiance Foundation to put up billboards promoting WhatAbortionReallyIs.com. The text-only billboards—which individually read "Abortion Is Lost Fatherhood," "Abortion Is Regret," "Abortion Is Fake Health," "Abortion Is Systemic Racism," and "Abortion Is Fake Feminism"—were denied.

Outfront Vice President Patrick J. Smith wrote in an email, "These are not going to be approved. We find them to be in the nature of *attack ads* and to be unnecessarily provocative and insensitive."[12] It is clear some in the media were not only suppressing the voices of Black pro-lifers but were censoring their messages as well.

Planned Parenthood's messaging, however, was gaining traction and becoming the main source of condemnation used to suppress pro-life voices. Their messaging also included changing the truth of their eugenic beginnings while camouflaging their population control intent. Until very recently, they went to great lengths not only to deny the eugenic foundation of their organization but to re-imagine Sanger as a "visionary social reformer."[13] The Negro Project, which they claim ended in 1942, "was designed to serve African Americans in the rural South. The advisory council called it a 'unique experiment in race-building and humanitarian service to a race subjected to discrimination, hardship, and segregation.'"[14] Though they acknowledged Sanger's eugenic beliefs, they downplayed the influence of her ideology while simultaneously attacking those activists considered to be "anti-family planning," stating: "Planned Parenthood Federation of America finds these views objectionable and outmoded. Nevertheless, anti-family planning activists continue to attack Sanger, who has been dead for nearly 40 years, because she is an easier target than the unassailable reputation of PPFA and the contemporary family planning movement."[15] Abortion apologists followed their lead, declaring pro-life advocates racists for pointing out the targeting and negative treatment of Black women.[16]

On occasion, abortion defenders fabricate narratives to promote the idea that pro-lifers are casting blame on Black women by pointing out the disparity in the numbers:

> Black women are blamed for a litany of ills that plague our community, and we're constantly disrespected for the choices we make regarding our bodies. On the one hand, a Black woman who goes through with an unwanted pregnancy and ends up having to use social services is shamed for being irresponsible and "leeching" off the system. On the other, a Black woman who makes the decision to terminate a pregnancy when they know having a child isn't the best idea can be shamed for endangering the future of her race.[17]

Their idea of truth is used to demonize the pro-life movement, declaring, "Pro-lifers always love to bring up the black abortion rate, claiming they are all for racial equality. Yet when black people are killed by police, the pro-life movement is silent. This proves their true intentions: not saving black lives, but controlling black women."[18] The real truth here is that pro-lifers are for racial equality but do not deflect to other social justice issues to assign blame to the Black woman. In fact, if blame and shame are assigned, it is almost always the abortion defenders who are doing so in efforts to make it appear as if it is the pro-life community doing so.

Abortion apologists also attack the pro-life movement for comparing abortion to slavery. Pro-life defenders sometimes argue that the same principles used by the Supreme Court to deny citizenship and personhood to Dred Scott were used in the *Roe* decision to deny personhood to the baby in utero. Some even believe the Court left the door open to overturning *Roe* on the basis of the Fourteenth Amendment (which was passed to abolish slavery), because if the personhood of preborn babies could be adequately proven, they would be protected under the Amendment.[19] However, as they have done with other pro-life arguments, abortion apologists try to use this line of reasoning against their opponents. They claim, "When slavery was legal, forcing slave women to get pregnant and give birth was very common. Pro-lifers compare abortion to slavery, but what they are doing is much more comparable to slavery."[20] Planned Parenthood gleefully agrees with and promotes these narratives and the idea of bodily autonomy that denies the personhood of the child in favor of the woman's right of self-determination.[21]

Capitalizing on Racial Injustice

Not too long after the horrific death of George Floyd on May 25, 2020, Planned Parenthood affiliates began issuing statements of solidarity with the Black community, declaring that the deaths of Black men and women at the hands of Caucasian policemen "must be answered with swift justice and reformative action. They, like so many before them, died because of racist violence or police brutality, which are often one and the same. They died because of the systemic racism that festers within our nation and pervades our country's police departments."[22]

Less than a month later, on June 18, 2020, defenders of Planned Parenthood again were caught off-guard when more than three hundred current and former employees of the organization publicly declared "Planned Parenthood was founded by a racist, white woman. That is a part of history that cannot be changed."[23] These employees began making the argument that Planned Parenthood was and is a bastion of the systemic racism they claimed the pro-life community represents. A month later, July 21, 2020, the president of the board of the New York affiliate went further, stating, "The removal of Margaret Sanger's name from our building is both a necessary and overdue step to reckon with our legacy and acknowledge Planned

Parenthood's contributions to historical reproductive harm within communities of color."[24] Never before had any abortion organization acknowledged causing harm to women of color.

Once New York opened the door, affiliates across the nation began confessing their own racist behaviors toward their Black employees. One affiliate, in owning their long-term racist behavior, said, "We must confront how white supremacy of the past *and present* continue in the institutions we are a part of today—*including our own organization*."[25] One Virginia Planned Parenthood, which had used the Black infant mortality rate to justify construction of a third surgical room in their facility, released a statement, part of which read, "We also acknowledge our past and our present participation in white supremacy and are committed to stopping, learning, growing and living our values through the hard and uncomfortable work of progress."[26]

Yet none of the facilities were truly turning away from their eugenic practices. Instead, they continue using civil rights rhetoric to downplay the systemic racism found throughout their organization. Central Coast Planned Parenthood, even while pretending to repent of their behaviors that contributed to a discriminatory environment, could not resist projecting the blame back onto the pro-life community. They said,

> Our commitment to racial justice also means calling out columnists and organizations who misuse and abuse the history around Sanger's complicated legacy to shame people, often specifically Black women, for seeking sexual and reproductive health care at Planned Parenthood health centers.
>
> Co-opting the Movement for Black Lives and expressing false concern for Black communities while seeking to

> eliminate people's access to safe, legal abortion is disgraceful. It infantilizes Black women by assuming they are incapable of making their own decisions about their bodies and families.[27]

Not one of the affiliates acknowledged the increasing number of injuries and deaths of Black and Latina women at the hands of Planned Parenthood's Caucasian abortionists.

Having mastered the art of projection, Planned Parenthood has used the Black Lives Matter organization to further their interests in maintaining a pipeline of Black women of childbearing age into their facilities. They make claims they are standing with those who died at the hands of White policemen, mixing in their ideas designed to maintain the fallacy of fighting for Black women: "The fundamental right to bodily autonomy—the belief that every person should be safe and free in their body—guides Planned Parenthood's work and our fight for reproductive freedom. State-sanctioned violence makes the promise of freedom unattainable for Black people in this country—that includes reproductive freedom"—as if abortion restrictions and police shootings were identical.[28]

The Negro Project's Trail of Pain

There comes a point, however, when projection becomes a mirror. Today, America can see that just as the knee of Derek Chauvin cut off the life of George Floyd, so the knees of Planned Parenthood and other abortionists rest on the necks of Black babies and are increasingly cutting off the breath of their mothers. One recent example is the death of Tia Parks in 2019 at Preterm, an abortion center in a Black neighborhood of Cleveland, Ohio—the very abortion facility that has posted billboards calling abortion sacred and a blessing. Tia was pregnant with twins, one of which was in her fallopian tube, and the center failed to detect it. She left the facility in intense pain believing she had a successful abortion. She died of a heart attack the day afterward when her fallopian tube ruptured.[29] Preterm, a sham of a reproductive healthcare center, failed to conduct a complete examination to determine if there were conditions that would complicate her surgery, even though she presented in a high-risk category (Tia was considered obese).

The trail of injured women across the nation know abortion is not safe. As revealed by Operation Rescue, a leading pro-life Christian activist organization, the number of documented medical emergencies has increased over the last five years. America has no idea how many of those women later die, because the abortion industry has blocked the accurate recording of such data. In 2019, there were one hundred documented cases of injury of varying degrees. Fifty-one of those cases happened at a Planned Parenthood, thirteen of which occurred at the flagship facility in New York formerly known as the Margaret Sanger Center. The center in St. Louis has sent seventy-five women to the hospital since 2009. And within sixty days of opening a new facility in Fairview Heights, Illinois, the abortionists (most of whom had worked at the St. Louis facility just a few miles away) sent another woman to the hospital—yet more evidence of the less-than-safe, substandard care abortionists provide.[30]

The masters of projection have made it appear that the pro-life community does not care about women, but, as has been the case for decades, it is the abortion industry that cares little for women. One of the more horrifying examples of their lack of care is the picture of an eighty-year-old abortionist, unable to move without a walker, entering an abortion center in Baton Rouge, Louisiana.[31] It is difficult to comprehend how such a person could be qualified to perform abortions. Sometimes abortion doctors are simply unreachable when their patients need them most. When twenty-nine-year-old Jennifer Morbelli experienced complications after her late term abortion (at 33 weeks), abortionist LeRoy Carhart was nowhere to be found. Neither employees in his clinic nor emergency room personnel were able to contact him, leaving the emergency room staff in the dark about any treatment she may have been provided. Sadly, Jennifer died.[32]

Battling with Pregnancy Centers

Any attempts to provide women with resources to choose life are objected to, strenuously, by the abortion industry. Pro-abortion organizations band together to stop life-affirming assistance to abortion-minded and determined women, taking steps to make sure they think abortion is the only choice. In the winter of 2011, members of the National Black Pro-life Coalition were invited to New York City to rally with local pastors and clergy against a recently introduced bill to require pregnancy centers to post notices disclosing whether they offered abortion services.[33] Led by City Council Chairwoman Christina Quinn, supporters of the bill labeled their efforts as a demand for truth in advertising. Focusing on whether there was a physician on staff to perform the pregnancy test or ultrasound, the bill sought to cast the pregnancy centers as fake clinics. The real impetus behind the bill was to stop women at the door of the center so they would not obtain a free pregnancy test and/or ultrasound, and would instead go to one of the abortion centers to which the pregnancy center was demanded to refer them.

The pregnancy center movement began as a volunteer effort to help expectant moms who choose life by providing resources to help throughout their pregnancy and birth, including diapers, maternity clothing, baby clothing, car seats, and other equipment needed for a newborn. In their effort to place real choice before women that was based on science and not emotion, pregnancy centers began offering free pregnancy tests and ultrasounds. Counselors were and are available to help women understand the ins and outs of a pregnancy, including fetal development and the physical and psychological impact of abortion. In addition, as the need was identified, pregnancy centers began offering abortion recovery to women, men, and families for healing from the trauma of abortion and broken relationships. These services seemed to create outrage among defenders of abortion, who began the effort to force pregnancy centers to post notices that not only referred for abortions but also stated abortions were not provided on their premises.

The New York City rally resulted in the formation of pastoral and clergy groups committed to standing against abortion in the city. This became an urgent charge once they realized that New York City was aborting more babies than were born alive.[34] While the rally activated the clergy network who are standing against abortion, it did not stop the bill from being passed. It took the engagement of Alliance Defending Freedom, a nonprofit organization that defends the sanctity of life, to take the matter to court in order to prevent what many believed to be a clear infringement on First Amendment rights.

NARAL Prochoice America has taken their ploy of attacking pregnancy centers for false advertising across the nation. A recent example is the introduction of a bill in Connecticut to prohibit "'deceptive advertising' practices by limited services pregnancy centers."[35] Though unable to produce actual clients to testify that they were misled by the pregnancy centers, NARAL has had the bill introduced three times.[36] Pregnancy centers were able to produce documentation of client satisfaction, with some rated as high as 95 percent satisfied. But this documentation did not deter the efforts of abortion defenders to prevent women from receiving help.

Conclusion

The abortion industry's disguised attacks against Black women and their babies are seemingly endless. The disguise has hidden the real facts from the eyes of average Americans, facts such as the location of the majority of abortion clinics. Seventy-eight percent of Planned Parenthood's surgical facilities are in or near Black and Latino communities, while *80 percent of their facilities that are 10,000 square feet or larger are in Black neighborhoods*.[37]

The manner in which Planned Parenthood and other abortion providers operate their services is having an adverse impact on Black women and babies. That negative impact is a violation of the Civil Rights Act of 1964. Federally assisted programs do not have the liberty to target a group based on skin color. Yet abortion is being used as an instrument of population control, just as Justice Ruth Bader Ginsburg revealed in her 2009 *New York Times Magazine* interview.[38] The abortion industry's marketing, however, has been successful in obfuscating its own impact on population control. When looking at the actual numbers, we find *abortion is the leading cause of death in the Black community*, taking the lives of more Blacks than the next seven leading causes of death combined.

Abortion is not safe despite the number of times its defenders say it is. Unfortunately, it is almost impossible to determine the number of injuries, whether psychological or physical, because the data is not collected. Women are dying and being injured while the industry moves toward allowing women to self-abort through RU-486 and similar pills. The physical and psychological risk to the woman increases in the cases where women use RU-486 and other pills to self-abort, but that risk is downplayed in favor of keeping abortion legal at all costs.

No matter how many Black leaders are groomed by Planned Parenthood and other pro-choice organizations to peddle abortion through their influence, the facts remain the same and the numbers do not lie. Abortion is having a holocaustic impact, especially in the Black community, which proportionally is abortion's number one customer.

The pro-life community is the last line of protection for women and girls who are abortion-minded and determined. The sidewalk counselors who see the destruction firsthand every day, the legislators who dare to take a stand and sponsor legislation to protect women and babies in the womb, the pro-life organizations that lobby for life at the state and national levels, the pregnancy centers that reach out hands of help and hope—these are all protectors to be celebrated. Like the abolitionists who fought and stood against slavery, members of the pro-life community are a shield of protection working in and for the Black community.

Acknowledgments

A project like this requires the support of many to see the light of day. We are grateful for all the prayers and partnerships we have benefited from throughout the planning and production processes, especially of those behind the scenes.

Thanks are due to the team at Moody Publishers, especially Bryan Litfin and Pam Pugh, for believing in and investing in this project. Bryan's enthusiasm for this project has been evident since day one. It was his leadership and encouragement that guided the book from the starting gate to the finish line. Pam provided expert input on matters of rhetoric, style, annotations, and various other necessary details, all of which improved the volume tremendously. Her careful editorial eye and good judgment saved us from not a few mistakes.

We are also grateful to our team of authors for their contributions not only to this volume but to the larger aims of the pro-life movement. It has been a great privilege to work with such an amazing lineup of lawyers, theologians, physicians, activists, and ministry leaders. Without their varied expertise and unwavering conviction, this project would not have been completed.

We are thankful for the encouragement and resources of our home institutions—Biola University (Jeanette); Moody Bible

Institute and Compass Bible Institute (John). Their shared vision to see the gospel impact real lives helped inspire this book.

We also owe a huge word of thanks to our spouses, Christin Goodrich and Nick Pifer. They have supported our respective scholarly interests for many years. We are very blessed to have them in our corner.

Finally, we are grateful for the *love*—indeed, for the very *lives*—of our respective sons, Justin Dylan Goodrich and Brantley John Pifer.

John: Justin, now eleven years old, has been a model of endless passion, perseverance, and playfulness, especially during some very difficult years impacted by COVID-19 and other family health crises. It is humbling to watch him grow into a young man who cares deeply about the well-being of others, not least the unborn. I am so very proud of him.

Jeanette: This volume got underway when Brantley was only a prayer. After trying to conceive for three years, suffering one miscarriage, and finally being told that our chances to conceive were essentially impossible, the Lord demonstrated once again that *He is the God of the impossible* (Luke 18:27). My work on this volume in the midst of all of this was accompanied with much emotion as well as conviction to fight ardently for the plight of millions of unborn children. As it turned out, it wasn't until the manuscript was completed that Brantley was conceived, and he is due roughly six weeks before this book will be in print. He is our gift from God, whose life we trust will exemplify his namesake—that he will live by the sword of the Spirit and carry within him a fire for the Lord.

We dedicate this volume to our little boys—to Justin and to Brantley. Your beautiful young lives are a blessing beyond words. Our prayer and our confidence is that the Lord will use you both mightily for His kingdom purposes.

Notes

Introduction: A Call for Compassionate Engagement

1. The aggregate data suggest that the number of abortions in the United States remains close to a million per year. While the number of annual abortions has dropped considerably over the past several decades, an increase was reported in 2018, perhaps due to the rise in chemical abortions. Unfortunately, the most reliable reporting is still very incomplete and contradictory. This is due to a number of factors, including the voluntary nature of state reporting (e.g., California doesn't report abortion data). See, e.g., Rachel K. Jones, Elizabeth Witwer, and Jenna Jerman, "Abortion Incidence and Service Availability in the United States, 2017," Guttmacher Institute, https://www.guttmacher.org/report/abortion-incidence-service-availability-us-2017; Tessa Longbons, "New Abortion Trends in the United States: A First Look," Charlotte Lozier Institute, September 22, 2020, https://lozierinstitute.org/new-abortion-trends-in-the-united-states-a-first-look/; Katherine Kortsmit et al., "Abortion Surveillance—United States, 2018," *Surveillance Summaries* 69.7 (2020): 1–29, https://www.cdc.gov/mmwr/volumes/69/ss/ss6907a1.htm.
2. James Davison Hunter, *Culture Wars: The Struggle to Define America* (New York: Basic Books, 1991), 42.
3. Ibid.
4. "Morality of Abortion, 2018–2020 Demographic Tables," Gallup, https://news.gallup.com/poll/244625/morality-abortion-2018-demographic-tables.aspx.
5. Ryan T. Anderson, "Religious Liberty Isn't Enough: Cultural Conservatives Also Need to Defend Our Views, Which Are Scientifically Sound and Popular," *Wall Street Journal*, https://www.wsj.com/articles/religious-liberty-isnt-enough-11612125595.
6. Admittedly, while this book models the way to speak about abortion in a healthy tone, it does not instruct the reader about how to do that. For such a helpful "how to" book, see Stephanie Gray, *Love Unleashes Life: Abortion and the Art of Communicating Truth* (Toronto: Life Cycle, 2015).

Chapter 1: A More Excellent Way: Moral Decision-Making beyond Government Law

1. Rob Reiner et al., *A Few Good Men* (motion picture), United States: Columbia Pictures, 1992.
2. Rebecca Todd Peters, *Trust Women: A Progressive Christian Argument for Reproductive Justice* (Boston: Beacon, 2018), 138 (some emphasis added).
3. Tom D. Campbell, *The Legal Theory of Ethical Positivism*, Applied Legal Philosophy (New York: Routledge, 2016), 1: "In legal theory, Legal Positivism is generally taken to be the view that the concept of law can be elucidated without reference to morality, and that it is the duty of judges to determine the content of and apply the law without recourse to moral judgments."
4. Scott B. Rae, *Moral Choices: An Introduction to Ethics*, 4th ed. (Grand Rapids: Zondervan Academic, 2018), 23 (emphasis in original).
5. Deni Elliott, "'Can' Does Not Equal 'Should': Distinguishing Ethics from Law," *Student Press Law Center Report* 6.2 (Spring 1985): 3–5.
6. Rae, *Moral Choices*, 24.
7. Alan J. Hawkins and Heather Smith, "National Survey Reveals Generation Differences in Consensual Nonmonogamy," Institute for Family Studies, September 11, 2019, https://ifstudies.org/blog/national-survey-reveals-generational-differences-in-consensual-nonmonogamy-.
8. Rae, *Moral Choices*, 53.
9. Ibid., 54.
10. Michael Gorman surveys evidence from antiquity and concludes that while Greek and Roman society showed little concern for the unborn, early Judaism and Christianity agreed about the immorality of abortion (*Abortion and the Early Church: Christian, Jewish and Pagan Attitudes in the Greco-Roman World* [Downers Grove, IL: InterVarsity Press, 1982]).
11. "Morality of Abortion, 2018–2020 Demographic Tables," Gallup, https://news.gallup.com/poll/244625/morality-abortion-2018-demographic-tables.aspx.
12. This syllogism is adapted from Francis J. Beckwith, *Defending Life: A Moral and Legal Case against Abortion Choice* (Cambridge: Cambridge University Press, 2007), xii.
13. Robert Young, "What Is So Wrong with Killing People?," *Philosophy* 54 (1979): 515–28, at 519: "What makes killing another human being wrong on occasions is its character as an irrevocable, maximally unjust prevention of the realization either of the victim's life-purposes or of such life-purposes as the victim may reasonably have been expected to resume or to come to have."
14. Robert J. Spitzer, *Healing the Culture: A Commonsense Philosophy of Happiness, Freedom and the Life Issues* (San Francisco: Ignatius, 2000), 241.
15. Carol Sanger, *About Abortion: Terminating Pregnancy in Twenty-First Century America* (Cambridge: The Belknap Press of Harvard University Press, 2017), 23.
16. Brian Dale, *Fertilization: The Beginning of Life* (Cambridge: Cambridge

University Press, 2018), ix (emphasis added).

17. Samuel Webster and Rhiannon de Wreede, *Embryology at a Glance*, 2nd ed. (Oxford: Wiley Blackwell, 2016), 2.
18. Ronan O'Rahilly and Fabiola Müller, *Human Embryology and Teratology*, 3rd ed. (New York: Wiley-Liss, 2001), 8 (emphasis in original).
19. For additional sources linking fertilization to the beginning of life, see the 44 quotations from medical textbooks and peer-reviewed scientific literature (published 2001–2016) compiled by Maureen Condic at https://bdfund.org/wp-content/uploads/2016/05/Condic-Sources-Embryology.pdf-old.
20. Steven Andrew Jacobs, "Balancing Abortion Right and Fetal Rights: A Mixed Methods Mediation of the U.S. Abortion Debate" (PhD diss., University of Chicago, 2019), 250.
21. Ibid.
22. John Janez Miklavcic and Paul Flaman, "Personhood Status of the Human Zygote, Embryo, Fetus," *Linacre Quarterly* 84 (2017): 130–44, https://doi.org/10.1080/00243639.2017.1299896; Christopher Kaczor, *The Ethics of Abortion: Women's Rights, Human Life, and the Question of Justice* (New York: Routledge, 2011).
23. Thomas R. Schreiner, *Galatians*, Zondervan Exegetical Commentary on the New Testament (Grand Rapids: Zondervan, 2010), 360. David deSilva says similarly: "As Christ takes shape in one by means of the working of the Spirit (2:20; 4:19), one becomes a person who similarly loves and serves as Christ did" (*The Letter to the Galatians*, New International Commentary on the New Testament [Grand Rapids: Eerdmans, 2018], 485).
24. Peters, *Trust Women*, 138 (emphasis added).

Chapter 2: *Roe v. Wade*: Destined for the Dustbin

1. Ruth Bader Ginsburg, "Some Thoughts on Autonomy and Equality in Relation to *Roe v. Wade*," *North Carolina Law Review* 63.2 (1985): 375–86, at 385–86, https://scholarship.law.unc.edu/cgi/viewcontent.cgi?article=2961&context=nclr.
2. John Hart Ely, "The Wages of Crying Wolf: A Comment on *Roe v. Wade*," *Yale Law Journal* 82 (1973): 920–49, at 935–37, 947, https://digitalcommons.law.yale.edu/cgi/viewcontent.cgi?article=6179&context=ylj.
3. Laurence H. Tribe, "The Supreme Court, 1972 Term—Foreword: Toward a Model of Roles in the Due Process of Life and Law," *Harvard Law Review* 87.1 (1973): 1–53, at 7, https://www.jstor.org/stable/1339866?origin=crossref.
4. Mark V. Tushnet, "Following the Rules Law Down: A Critique of Interpretivism and Neutral Principles," *Harvard Law Review* 96.4 (1983): 781–827, at 820, https://doi.org/10.2307/1340904.
5. Kermit Roosevelt, "Shaky Basis for a Constitutional 'Right'," *Washington Post* (January 22, 2003), https://www.washingtonpost.com/archive/opinions/2003/01/22/shaky-basis-for-a-constitutional-right/dd30d42e-188d-42f6-

8fb2-b935394e63aa/.

6. Jeffrey Rosen, "Why We'd Be Better off Without *Roe*: Worst Choice," *The New Republic* (February 19, 2003), https://web.archive.org/web/20030309173117/http://www.tnr.com/doc.mhtml?i=20030224&s=rosen022403.
7. John Keown, "Back to the Future of Abortion Law: *Roe*'s Rejection of America's History and Traditions," *Issues in Law and Medicine* 22.1 (2006): 3–37, at 5, https://static1.squarespace.com/static/55d78cd0e4b00365e96a9dcc/t/59e110cfcd39c37ad08b742f/1507922128972/Back+to+the+Future+of+Abortion+Law.pdf.
8. William Blackstone, *Commentaries on the Laws of England* (Oxford: Clarendon, 1768), 1:129.
9. See, e.g., *Planned Parenthood of Central Missouri v. Danforth*, 428 U.S. 52, 99 (1976) (J. White).
10. Available at https://aul.org/publications/unsafe/.
11. Helen M. Alvaré, "Abortion, Sexual Markets and the Law," in *Persons, Moral Worth, and Embryos: A Critical Analysis of Pro-Choice Arguments*, ed. Stephen Napier (New York: Springer, 2011), 255–79, at 256.
12. Ibid.
13. Mara Hvistendahl, *Unnatural Selection: Choosing Boys Over Girls, and the Consequences of a World Full of Men* (New York: Public Affairs, 2011).
14. Honorable Vince Chhabria, United States District Judge, *Roundup Products Liability Litigation* (2019).
15. Jose Russo and Irma H. Russo, "Susceptibility of the Mammary Gland to Carcinogenesis—II. Pregnancy Interruption as a Risk Factor in Tumor Incidence," *American Journal of Pathology* 100.2 (August 1980): 497–512, https://www.ncbi.nlm.nih.gov/pmc/articles/PMC1903536/pdf/amjpathol00228-0184.pdf.
16. Pierre Band et al., "Carcinogenic and Endocrine Disrupting Effects of Cigarette Smoke and Risk of Breast Cancer," *The Lancet* 360,9339 (Oct. 5, 2002): 1044–49, https://doi.org/10.1016/S0140-6736(02)11140-8.
17. J. R. Daling et al., "Risk of Breast Cancer Among Young Women: Relationship to Induced Abortion," *Journal of the National Cancer Institute* 21.2 (1994): 1584–92, https://doi.org/10.1093/jnci/86.21.1584.
18. Joel Brind et al., "Induced Abortion as an Independent Risk Factor for Breast Cancer: A Comprehensive Review and Meta-Analysis," *Journal of Epidemiology and Community Health* 50 (1996): 481–96, https://jech.bmj.com/content/jech/50/5/481.full.pdf.
19. See https://www.reelhouse.org/mightymotionpictures/hushfilm.
20. See the NIH video archives, https://videocast.nih.gov/watch=2258 (minute 29:25), or *Hush* at 39:50.
21. *Hush* at 48:48.
22. Dr. Freda Bush, in *Hush* at 1:05:01.
23. P. S. Shah and J. Zao, "Induced Termination of Pregnancy and Low Birthweight and Preterm Birth: A Systematic Review and Meta-Analyses," *British Journal of Obstetrics and Gynaecology* 116.11 (September 16, 2009): 1425–42, https://

obgyn.onlinelibrary.wiley.com/doi/pdf/10.1111/j.1471-0528.2009.02278.x.

24. Catherine Glenn Foster, "What a Flawed Study Ignores about Abortion Regrets," *Washington Examiner* (January 17, 2020), https://www.washingtonexaminer.com/opinion/op-eds/what-a-flawed-study-ignores-about-abortion-regrets.
25. Priscilla K. Coleman, "Abortion and Mental Health: Quantitative Synthesis and Analysis of Research Published 1995–2009," *British Journal of Psychiatry* 199.3 (2011): 180–86, https://www.cambridge.org/core/journals/the-british-journal-of-psychiatry/article/abortion-and-mental-health-quantitative-synthesis-and-analysis-of-research-published-19952009/E8D556AAE1C1D2F0F8B060B28BEE6C3D.
26. Brenda Major et al., "Mental Health and Abortion," 2008, https://www.apa.org/pi/women/programs/abortion/mental-health.pdf.
27. Aimee Murphy and Catherine Glenn Foster, "Restore the Heart," Rehumanize International and Americans United for Life, January 2020, https://aul.org/wp-content/uploads/2020/07/restore-the-heart-white-paper-web.pdf, 20.
28. For a lengthier summary, see the AUL legal memorandum: https://aul.org/wp-content/uploads/2020/08/2020-07-31-AUL-on-JMS-Disapointment-and-Opportunity.pdf.

Chapter 3: Made in God's Image: Personhood according to Scripture

1. Calum MacKellar, *The Image of God, Personhood and the Embryo* (London: SCM, 2017), 51.
2. E.g., René Descartes, John Locke, Immanuel Kant, and more recently Peter Singer and John Harris.
3. MacKellar, *The Image of God*, 59.
4. John D. Zizioulas, *Being as Communion: Studies in Personhood and the Church* (Crestwood, NY: St. Vladimir's Seminary Press, 1985), 27.
5. MacKellar, *The Image of God*, 63.
6. According to Gerhard von Rad: "It is correct to say that the verb *bara*, 'create,' contains the idea both of complete effortlessness and *creatio ex nihilo*, since it is never connected with any statement of the material. The hidden grandeur of this statement is that God is the Lord of the world" (*Genesis: A Commentary*, Old Testament Library [Philadelphia: Westminster, 1972], 49).
7. von Rad, *Genesis*, 57.
8. Maass, *ādhām*, *Theological Dictionary of the Old Testament*, ed. G. J. Botterweck et al. (Grand Rapids: Eerdmans, 1974), 1:75–87.
9. John Goldingay, *Biblical Theology: The God of the Christian Scriptures* (Downers Grove: IVP Academic, 2016), 173. This idea of being made in God's image occurs seven times in Scripture ("in his image," occurs in Gen. 1:26, 27; 9:6; 1 Cor. 11:7; "in his likeness" occurs in Gen. 1:26; 5:1; James 3:9). In other instances, Paul refers to humans being restored to the image of God through redemption in Christ Jesus (Col. 3:10; Eph. 4:24 and Acts 17:28–29—in Acts 17 the idea is present but the term is not).

10. von Rad, *Genesis*, 60.
11. H. Wildberger, "*ṣelem* image," in *Theological Lexicon of the Old Testament*, ed. Ernst Jenni and Claus Westermann, trans. Mark E. Biddle (Peabody, MA: Hendrickson, 1997), 1080–85.
12. Robert L. Saucy, "Theology of Human Nature," in *Christian Perspectives on Being Human: A Multidisciplinary Approach to Integration*, ed. J. P. Moreland and David M. Ciocchi (Grand Rapids: Baker, 1993), 20.
13. Saucy, "Theology of Human Nature," 20.
14. Ryan S. Peterson, *The Imago Dei as Human Identity: A Theological Interpretation*, JTISup 14 (Winona Lake, IN: Eisenbrauns, 2016).
15. Some pro-choice proponents criticize these kinds of appeals to poetic verses about life in the womb by those like me seeking to establish prenatal personhood. Margaret D. Kamitsuka, for example, asserts: "This attempt to prove biblically that an embryo is a predestined person is based on a dubious exegetical approach that extrapolates a universal theological claim from a handful of mostly poetic verses in the Hebrew Bible" (*Abortion and the Christian Tradition: A Pro-Choice Theological Ethic* [Louisville: Westminster John Knox, 2019], 50). Kamitsuka's general critique is unwarranted, for poetry is often used in the Bible as a worshipful expression of deep theological reflection. Poetry often employs figurative language, but this hardly means that nothing it conveys is literal, or even that figures of speech can't provide a window into the anthropological assumptions of the biblical authors. The use of poetry alone should therefore not constitute a decisive ruling out of the content being eloquently described.

    Nevertheless, for additional support we can look to the New Testament, to the calling and consecration of Paul, who appeals to God who "had set me apart before I was born, and who called me by his grace" (Gal. 1:15). This passage lies outside the genre of poetry and supports the argument that Scripture reveals instances of God's personal calling, care, and sovereign design of life from its earliest stages before birth. Indeed, the prophetic voices of Jeremiah and Isaiah, together with the apostle Paul, propound a theology of divine intention attributed to prenatal life. This divine calling is accompanied by an intimate knowledge of the person developing inside his mother's belly at the earliest stages.
16. The phrase "in the depths of the earth" is a metaphor for the deepest concealment, in this case the "hiddenness of the womb" (Derek Kidner, *Psalms 73–150: A Commentary*, TOTC [Downers Grove, IL: InterVarsity Press, 1973], 466; J. Clinton McCann, Jr., *The Book of Psalms: Introduction, Commentary, and Reflections*, NIB IV (Nashville: Abingdon, 1996), 1236.
17. F. Brown, S. R. Driver & C. A. Briggs, *Enhanced Brown-Driver-Briggs Hebrew and English Lexicon* (Oxford: Clarendon Press, 1977), 166. Cf. Lexham English Bible.
18. John Goldingay, *Psalms 90–150*, Baker Commentary on the Old Testament Wisdom and Psalms (Grand Rapids: Baker, 2008), 634.
19. John Jefferson Davis, "The Moral Status of the Embryonic Human: Religious

Perspectives," *Ethics & Medicine* 22:1 (2006): 9–21, at 11.

20. The early Church Fathers such as Clement, Tertullian, and Chrysostom read this text with the understanding that the embryos in both Elizabeth and in Mary were alive and personal. Clement of Alexandria *Prophetic Eclogues* 41 and 48–49; Tertullian *De anima* 26.4; Chrysostom *Homily 24 on the Epistle to the Romans.*
21. Davis, "The Moral Status of the Embryonic Human," 15.
22. John Jefferson Davis, *Evangelical Ethics: Issues Facing the Church Today* (Phillipsburg, NJ: P&R Publishing, 1985), 150.
23. The Hebrew text uses the plural form for children here. This is probably to indicate the possibility that a mother in such a scenario could be carrying more than one child; however, the text naturally applies to situations in which the mother is carrying only one child. For ease of prose, I will discuss the issue in view of a singular translation.
24. Scholars who hold to this translation generally do so on the basis of parallels found in other Ancient Near Eastern literature. For example, one is hard-pressed to find examples of a viable premature birth when a pregnant woman is struck in extrabiblical legal codes (John Makujina, "The Semantics of *Yatsa* in Exodus 21:22: Reassessing the Variables that Determine Meaning," *BBR* 23:3 [2013]: 305–21, at 306).
25. Brown, Driver & Briggs, *Enhanced Brown-Driver-Briggs Hebrew and English Lexicon.*
26. The same verb is also used to refer to animals in Genesis 31:38 and Job 21:10, and in 2 Kings 2:19, 21 and Malachi 3:11 it refers to land and plants that do not yield mature fruit.
27. Makujina, "Semantics of *Yatsa*," 306.
28. Gen. 25:25, 26; 38:28, 29, 30; Ex. 21:22; Num. 12:12; Deut. 28:57; Jer. 1:5; 20:18; Job 1:21; 3:11; 10:18; 38:8, 29; Eccl. 5:14. Outside the Pentateuch, the verb is often used in poetic ways rather than explicit birth narratives. For example, Job 1:21 and Ecclesiastes 5:14 describe the nakedness of a baby when it enters the world and its nakedness when it leaves this world. For more discussion on these texts, see Makujina, "The Semantics of *Yatsa*," 308–09.
29. See, e.g., Gen. 35:16–18 and 1 Sam. 4:19–20 for additional difficult births. Cf. Makujina, "The Semantics of *Yatsa*," 311–12.
30. Cf. also Job 3:11 where Job speaks hypothetically of dying at birth. Here also the verb is modified with some form of the verb *muth* meaning "to die."
31. Richard M. Davidson, *Flame of Yahweh: Sexuality in the Old Testament* (Peabody, MA: Hendrickson, 2007), 496; Makujina, "The Semantics of *Yatsa*," 313.
32. Davidson, *Flame of Yahweh*, 496.
33. Cf. the election of Jacob in the womb of Rebekah (Gen. 25:23); David confesses he was a sinner from the time of his conception (Ps. 51:5); John the Baptist was filled with the Holy Spirit in his mother's womb (Luke 1:15). Note that often names were divinely given before birth (e.g., Ishmael [Gen. 16:11]; John the Baptist [Luke 1:13], Jesus [Matt. 1:21]). Davis notes: "These divinely appointed names are unmistakable indications that God viewed these individuals as *persons*

before birth, from the very beginning of the human life cycle, inasmuch as a personal name is the crucial marker of human personal status" ("The Moral Status of the Embryonic Human," 14).

34. Davis, "The Moral Status of the Embryonic Human," 13.

Chapter 4: More Than the Sum of Its Parts: Philosophical Reflections on Human Personhood

1. For a more extended discussion of the distinction between substances and property things, see J. P. Moreland and Scott B. Rae, *Body and Soul: Human Nature and the Crisis in Ethics* (Downers Grove, IL: IVP Academic, 2000), 49–86.
2. For further information on these various markers for personhood, see Francis J. Beckwith, *Defending Life: A Moral and Legal Case against Abortion Choice* (Cambridge: Cambridge University Press, 2007).
3. Bonnie Steinbock, *Life Before Birth: The Moral and Legal Status of Embryos and Fetuses,* 2nd ed. (Oxford: Oxford University Press, 2011).
4. For discussion of this view, see Alberto Giubilini and Francesca Minerva, "After-Birth Abortion: Why Should the Baby Live?" *Journal of Medical Ethics* 39.5 (2013): 261–63; Peter Singer, *Practical Ethics* (Cambridge: Cambridge University Press, 1979). For critique, see Gordon R. Preece, ed., *Rethinking Peter Singer: A Christian Critique* (Downers Grove, IL: InterVarsity Press, 2002).
5. For further explanation of this view, see Mary Anne Warren, *Moral Status: Obligations to Persons and Other Living Things* (Oxford: Oxford University Press, 1997).
6. See Judith Jarvis Thomson, "A Defense of Abortion," *Philosophy and Public Affairs* 1 (1971): 47–66. For further critique, see Francis J. Beckwith, *Defending Life.*

Chapter 5: Knit Together in a Mother's Womb: The Biology of Prenatal Development

1. T. W. Sadler, *Langman's Medical Embryology,* 14th ed. (Philadelphia: Wolters Kluwer, 2019).
2. Ibid.
3. "Prenatal Form and Function—The Making of an Earth Suit," at Appendix A—Calculations (The Beat Goes On: Tracking the Total Number of Heart Beats During Pregnancy and Beyond), The Endowment for Human Development, https://www.ehd.org/dev_article_appendix.php.
4. "Shocking Video: Millions Dead," Life Dynamics Inc., https://youtu.be/ektNpslOUPM.
5. Planned Parenthood, https://www.plannedparenthood.org/learn/abortion/considering-abortion/what-facts-about-abortion-do-i-need-know.
6. "Can you see the products of the abortion (placenta, embryo, blood) and what should you do with them?" Aid Access, https://aidaccess.org/en/page/456/can-you-see-the-products-of-the-abortion-placenta-embryo-blood-and-what-shou.

7. "Person," Merriam-Webster Dictionary, https://www.merriam-webster.com/dictionary/person.
8. Ronan O'Rahilly and Fabiola Müller, *Developmental Stages in Human Embryos: Including a Revision of Streeter's "Horizons" and a Survey of the Carnegie Collection* (Washington, DC: Carnegie Institution of Washington, 637, 1987).
9. "Developmental Anatomy," National Museum of Health and Medicine, https://www.medicalmuseum.mil/?p=collections.hdac.anatomy.index.
10. Maureen L. Condic, "When Does Human Life Begin? The Scientific Evidence and Terminology Revisited," *University of St. Thomas Journal of Law and Public Policy* 8.1 (2013): 44–81; and idem, "A Scientific View of When Life Begins" (June 11, 2014), Charlotte Lozier Institute, https://lozierinstitute.org/a-scientific-view-of-when-life-begins/.
11. "For you created my inmost being; you knit me together in my mother's womb. I praise you because I am fearfully and wonderfully made; your works are wonderful, I know that full well. My frame was not hidden from you when I was made in the secret place, when I was woven together in the depths of the earth. Your eyes saw my unformed body; all the days ordained for me were written in your book before one of them came to be" (Ps. 139:13–16 NIV).
12. J. D. Watson and F. H. C. Crick, "A Structure of Deoxyribose Nucleic Acid," *Nature* 171 (1953): 737–78.
13. I. K. Suzuki et al., "Human-Specific *NOTCH2NL* Genes Expand Cortical Neurogenesis through Delta/Notch Regulation," *Cell* 173 (May 31, 2018): 1370–84, https://doi.org/10.1016/j.cell.2018.03.067. Also Ed Yong, "Searching for the Genes That Are Unique to Humans," October 13, 2015. Francis Collins, "Study Shows Genes Unique to Humans Tied to Bigger Brains," at *NIH Director's Blog*, June 5, 2021, https://directorsblog.nih.gov/2018/06/05/study-shows-genes-unique-to-humans-tied-to-bigger-brains/.
14. E. Bianconi et al., "An Estimation of the Number of Cells in the Human Body," *Annals of Human Biology* 40, no. 6 (2013): 463–71, https://doi.org/10.3109/03014460.2013.807878.
15. International Human Genome Sequencing Consortium, "Finishing the Euchromatic Sequence of the Human Genome," *Nature* 431 (2004): 931–45, https://doi.org/10.1038/nature03001.
16. J. Hirsch, "Uniqueness, Diversity, Similarity, Repeatability, and Heritability," *International Journal of Comparative Psychology* 17, no. 4 (2004): 304–14, https://escholarship.org/uc/item/1398d56t.
17. Ibid.
18. "Prenatal Form and Function—The Making of an Earth Suit," at Appendix A—Calculations (To the Sun and Back: Computing the Length of DNA in an Adult), The Endowment for Human Development, https://www.ehd.org/dev_article_appendix.php.
19. Ronan O'Rahilly and Fabiola Müller, *Human Embryology and Teratology*, 3rd ed. (New York: Wiley-Liss, 2001), 8.

20. Peter Singer, *Practical Ethics*, 3rd ed. (Cambridge: Cambridge University Press, 2011), 73.
21. Margaret Sanger, "The Pope's Position on Birth Control," January 27, 1932, in *The Selected Papers of Margaret Sanger—Volume 2: Birth Control Comes of Age, 1928–1939*, ed. Esther Katz et al. (Urbana, IL: University of Illinois Press, 2006), 150.
22. Steven Andrew Jacobs, "Balancing Abortion Right and Fetal Rights: A Mixed Methods Mediation of the U.S. Abortion Debate" (PhD diss., University of Chicago, 2019), 250, https://knowledge.uchicago.edu/record/1883?ln=en.
23. Media report: Steve Jacobs, "I Asked Thousands of Biologists When Life Begins. The Answer Wasn't Popular," *Quillette*, https://quillette.com/2019/10/16/i-asked-thousands-of-biologists-when-life-begins-the-answer-wasnt-popular/.
24. "Developmental Anatomy," National Museum of Health and Medicine, https://www.medicalmuseum.mil/?p=collections.hdac.anatomy.index.
25. O'Rahilly and Müller, *Human Embryology and Teratology*; 3rd ed.; and The Endowment for Human Development, https://www.ehd.org/prenatal-summary.php#fb38.
26. For helpful resources on the entire process of human embryonic and fetal development, see the Endowment for Human Development, https://www.ehd.org and the Biology of Prenatal Development DVD video; Contend Projects, https://contendprojects.org; M. A. Hill, Embryology, https://embryology.med.unsw.edu.au/embryology/index.php/Main_Page; T. W. Sadler, *Langman's Medical Embryology*, 14th ed. (Philadelphia: Wolters Kluwer, 2019); and Charlotte Lozier Institute, https://lozierinstitute.org/.
27. Lenore Pereira, "Congenital Viral Infection: Traversing the Uterine-Placental Interface," *Annual Review of Virology* 5, no. 1 (September 2018): 273–99, https://doi.org/10.1146/annurev-virology-092917-043236.
28. Gavin S. Dawe et al., "Cell Migration from Baby to Mother," *Cell Adhesion & Migration* 1, no. 1 (2007): 19–27, https://www.ncbi.nlm.nih.gov/pmc/articles/PMC2633676/pdf/cam0101_0019.pdf.
29. "Birth Defects—Data & Statistics," Centers for Disease Control and Prevention, https://www.cdc.gov/ncbddd/birthdefects/data.html; Alexander C. Egbe, "Birth Defects in the Newborn Population: Race and Ethnicity," *Pediatrics & Neonatology* 56.3 (2015): 183–88, https://doi.org/10.1016/j.pedneo.2014.10.002).
30. Colleen Malloy, Monique C. Wubbenhorst, and Tara Sander Lee, "The Perinatal Revolution," *Issues in Law and Medicine* 34, no. 1 (2019): 15–41, https://issuesinlawandmedicine.com/product/malloy-the-perinatal-revolution/.
31. Colleen Malloy, Congressional Testimony, 2016. https://www.judiciary.senate.gov/download/03-15-16-malloy-testimony; "Fact Sheet: Science of Fetal Pain," Charlotte Lozier Institute, https://lozierinstitute.org/fact-sheet-science-of-fetal-pain/.
32. Louisiana Health Law, Chapter 3. LA-RS 9 §121–§133, https://biotech.law.lsu.edu/cases/la/health/embryo_rs.htm.

33. Embryo Adoption Awareness Center, https://embryoadoption.org.
34. "National Embryo Donation Center Becomes First Embryo Adoption Program in the World to Mark 1,000-Birth Milestone," Christian NewsWire, http://christiannewswire.com/news/3610084562.html.
35. Ibid.

Chapter 6: Equal Protection for the Preborn: A Case for Prenatal Personhood according to the Fourteenth Amendment

1. This chapter is adapted from Joshua J. Craddock, "Protecting Prenatal Persons: Does the Fourteenth Amendment Prohibit Abortion?," *Harvard Journal of Law & Public Policy* 40, no. 2 (2017): 539–71, https://ssrn.com/abstract=2970761.
2. *Roe v. Wade,* 410 U.S. 113, 156 (1973).
3. Ibid., 158.
4. John Hart Ely, "The Wages of Crying Wolf: A Comment on *Roe v. Wade,*" *Yale Law Journal* 82, no. 5 (1973): 920–49.
5. See Robert A. Destro, "Abortion and the Constitution: The Need for a Life-Protective Amendment," *California Law Review* 63.5 (1975): 1250–1351, at 1278, https://doi.org/10.2307/3479846.
6. *Roe,* 410 U.S. at 156–57.
7. U.S. Const. amend. XIV, § 1.
8. UN General Assembly, "Universal Declaration of Human Rights," 217 (III) A, art. 6 (Paris, 1948), http://www.un.org/en/universal-declaration-human-rights/.
9. Nathan Schlueter, "Constitutional Persons: An Exchange on Abortion," *First Things,* January 2003, https://www.firstthings.com/article/2003/01/constitutional-persons-an-exchange-on-abortion.
10. The scientific and medical answer as to whether a prenatal life qualifies as a distinct human being had been available for over a century at the time of *Roe.* The *Roe* Court confused the scientifically and medically answerable question about when a new human organism's life begins with the ethical and legal question of whether that life possesses intrinsic value and demands protection. But since the scientific discoveries of the nineteenth century, disagreement has existed only over the latter question.
11. Schlueter, "Constitutional Persons."
12. E.g., "Person," in *A New Law Dictionary and Glossary,* A. M. Burrill (New York: John S. Voorhies, 1850): "A human being, considered as the subject of rights, as distinguished from a *thing.*" "Person," *The Law-Dictionary,* T. E. Tomlins, 1st Am. ed. (Philadelphia: R. H. Small, 1836): "A man or woman." "Person," *An American Dictionary of the English Language,* Noah Webster (New York: S. Converse, 1828): "An individual human being. . . . It is applied alike to a man, woman, or child."
13. "Person," *An American Dictionary of the English Language,* Noah Webster (Springfield, MA: G&C Merriam, 1864).

14. "Human," *An American Dictionary of the English Language* (1864). "Man" is in turn defined as, "An individual of the human race; a human being; a person" ("man," *An American Dictionary of the English Language* [1864]).
15. John D. Gorby, "The Right to an Abortion, the Scope of Fourteenth Amendment Personhood, and the Supreme Court's Birth Requirement," *Southern Illinois University Law Journal* 4 (1979): 1–36, at 23.
16. William Blackstone, *Commentaries on the Laws of England* (Oxford: Clarendon, 1768), 1:119.
17. Michael Stokes Paulsen, "The Plausibility of Personhood," *Ohio State Law Journal* 74 (2013): 13–74, at 26.
18. Blackstone, *Commentaries on the Laws of England,* 1:125.
19. Paulsen, "The Plausibility of Personhood," 28.
20. Intratextualism compares the uses of a term within a document to infer that term's meaning. Akhil Reed Amar, "Intratextualism," *Harvard Law Review* 112 (1999): 747–827.
21. Ibid, 792.
22. See *Roe,* 410 U.S. at 157; see also Amar, "Intratextualism," 792.
23. U.S. Const. amend. XIV, § 1.
24. Aliens, Indian natives, and even African slaves were generally considered persons, even though in most cases they were not citizens. See Paulsen, "The Plausibility of Personhood," 20. The term "person" has always been larger than the subset "citizen," and the Supreme Court's longstanding interpretation of the Fourteenth Amendment reflects that traditional understanding. See Plyler v. Doe, 457 U.S. 202, 212 (1982) (quoting *Yick Wo v. Hopkins,* 118 U.S. 356, 369 [1886]).
25. Paulsen, "The Plausibility of Personhood," 36.
26. Gorby, "The Right to an Abortion, the Scope of Fourteenth Amendment Personhood, and the Supreme Court's Birth Requirement," 15.
27. James S. Witherspoon, "Reexamining Roe: Nineteenth-Century Abortion Statutes and the Fourteenth Amendment," *St. Mary's Law Journal* 17 (1985): 29–71, at 48.
28. Ibid.
29. Ibid.
30. Robert M. Byrn, "An American Tragedy: The Supreme Court on Abortion," *Fordham Law Review* 41 (1972–1973): 807–62, at 861.
31. Ibid., 849.
32. Ibid., 819–20, quoting Sir Edward Coke, *The Third Part of the Institutes of the Laws of England: Concerning High Treason, and Other Pleas of the Crown, and Criminal Causes* (London: E. and R. Brooke, 1797), 50.
33. Byrn, "An American Tragedy," 824.
34. See *Roe,* 410 U.S. at 132–39.
35. John Keown, "Back to the Future of Abortion Law: Roe's Rejection of America's History and Traditions," *Issues in Law and Medicine* 22 (2006–2007): 3–37, at 6.
36. Byrn, "An American Tragedy," 825.

37. *Regina v. Wycherley*, 173 Eng. Rep. 486 (1838).
38. Thomas Percival and Chauncey D. Leake, *Percival's Medical Ethics* (New York: Ams Press, 1975 [1827]), 135–36.
39. 12 Trans. of the Am. Med. Assn. 76 (1859) (quoted in *Roe*, 410 U.S. at 141).
40. Ibid.
41. Byrn, "An American Tragedy," 836.
42. Keown, "Back to the Future of Abortion Law," 6.
43. Gorby, "The Right to an Abortion, the Scope of Fourteenth Amendment Personhood, and the Supreme Court's Birth Requirement," 15 (quoting *Mills v. Commonwealth*, 13 Pa. 631, 632–33 [1850]).
44. *Smith v. State*, 33 Me. 48 (1851).
45. Keown, "Back to the Future of Abortion Law," 27.
46. Ibid., Witherspoon, "Reexamining Roe," 33.
47. Keown, "Back to the Future of Abortion Law," 27.
48. Witherspoon, "Reexamining Roe," 48.
49. Ibid., 48–49.
50. Ibid., 40.
51. Ibid., 44. That some states did not treat abortion as murder does not indicate that the victim had less value or lacked personhood. Rather, it suggests the perpetrator was less culpable in some way, or that policy reasons dictated a lesser punishment.
52. Ibid., 42–44.
53. Ibid., 42–43.
54. Ibid., 61.
55. Ibid., 62.
56. Ibid., quoting 1867 Ohio Senate J. App. 233.
57. Ibid., quoting 1867 Ohio Senate J. App. 233.
58. Ibid., quoting 1867 Ohio Senate J. App. 233.
59. Ibid., 63, quoting 1867 Ohio Senate J. App. 233.
60. Ibid.
61. Ibid., 65.
62. Ibid., 65–69.
63. Ibid.
64. Byrn, "An American Tragedy," 813.
65. Cong. Globe, 39th Cong., 1st Sess. 2766 (1866).
66. Ibid.
67. Representative Thaddeus Stevens, Address at Bedford, Pa. (Sept. 4, 1866), in *Sacramento Daily Union*, Oct. 3, 1866, at 1.
68. Cong. Globe, 38th Cong., 1st Sess. 1753 (1864).
69. Representative John Bingham, Address at Bowerston, Ohio (Aug. 24, 1866), in Cin. Com., *The Constitutional Amendment Discussed by Its Author*, Sept. 11, 1866, at 19.
70. Cong. Globe, 40th Cong., 2nd Sess. 514–15 (1868) (emphasis added).
71. Destro, "Abortion and the Constitution," 1289.

72. Paulsen, "The Plausibility of Personhood," 51.
73. *United States v. Palmer*, 16 U.S. 610, 631–32 (1818).
74. *Conn. General Life Ins. Co. v. Johnson*, 303 U.S. 77, 87 (1938) (Black, J., dissenting).
75. 109 U.S. 3 (1883).
76. 378 U.S. 226, 309–11 (1964) (Goldberg, J., concurring).
77. Charles E. Rice, "Overruling Roe v. Wade: An Analysis of the Proposed Constitutional Amendments," *Boston College Industrial and Commercial Law Review* 15.2 (1973): 307–41, at 336.
78. See *Reitman v. Mulkey*, 387 U.S. 369 (1967); see also John E. Archibold, "Re-Examine State Abortion Law, Opponent Urges," *Denver Post*, July 7, 1968 (applying *Reitman* to the abortion context). Typically, "a State's failure to protect an individual against private violence [does] not constitute a violation of the Due Process Clause." Charles I. Lugosi, "Conforming to the Rule of Law: When Person and Human Being Finally Mean the Same Thing in Fourteenth Amendment Jurisprudence," *Issues in Law and Medicine* 22 (2006–2007): 119–303, at 291 (citing *DeShaney v. Winnebago Cty*. Dep't of Soc. Serv., 489 U.S. 189 [1989]). Nevertheless, the *DeShaney* Court qualified its holding by recognizing that "the State may not, of course, selectively deny its protective services to certain disfavored minorities without violating the Equal Protection Clause," 489 U.S. at 197 n. 3 (citing *Yick Wo*, 118 U.S. 356). The Court's reference to *Yick Wo* is telling. In that case, which extended Fourteenth Amendment guarantees to all persons (not just citizens), the Court condemned the "unjust and . . . discriminat[ory]" exercise of "purely personal and arbitrary power" over weak and disfavored groups (*Yick Wo*, 118 U.S. at 369–70). Thus, based on these precedents, if states were to systematically deny human beings *in utero* the protection of generally applicable laws against homicide, it would violate equal protection.
79. See, e.g., *Raleigh Fitkin-Paul Mem'l Hosp. v. Anderson*, 201 A.2d 537 (N.J. 1964), cert. denied 377 U.S. 985 (1964).
80. Ibid. at 538.
81. Gregory J. Roden, "Unborn Children as Constitutional Persons," *Issues in Law & Medicine* 25 (2010): 185–273, at 186.
82. U.S. Const. amend. XIV, § 5.
83. U.S. Const. art. II, § 3.

Chapter 7: Whose Body? The Illusion of Autonomy

1. Jane Doe, "There Just Wasn't Room in Our Lives Now for Another Baby," *New York Times*, May 14, 1976, https://www.nytimes.com/1976/05/14/archives/there-just-wasnt-room-in-our-lives-now-for-another-baby.html.
2. James Stacey Taylor, "Autonomy," Encyclopædia Britannica (Encyclopædia Britannica, Inc., June 20, 2017), https://www.britannica.com/topic/autonomy.
3. Tom L. Beauchamp and James F. Childress, *Principles of Biomedical Ethics*, 8th ed. (Oxford: Oxford University Press, 2019).

4. Cf. Daniel Callahan, "When Self-Determination Runs Amok," *The Hastings Center Report* 22.2 (March/April 1992): 51–55, at 52, https://doi.org/10.2307/3562566; available at https://users.manchester.edu/Facstaff/SSNaragon/Online/texts/235/Callahan,%20Self-Determination.pdf.
5. Michelle Llamas, "Black Box Warnings—Fast-Tracked Drugs & Increased Use," Drugwatch.com, April 20, 2020, https://www.drugwatch.com/fda/black-box-warnings/.
6. "iPLEDGE: Safety Notice," ipledgeprogram.com, 2016, https://www.ipledgeprogram.com/iPledgeUI/home.u.
7. "Rising Cost of OB/GYN Medical Malpractice Insurance," eQuoteMD, March 8, 2016, https://equotemd.com/blog/obgyn-medical-malpractice-insurance/.
8. I. B. Van den Veyver, "Prenatal Genetic Testing and Screening," in *Chimerism,* ed. N. Draper (New York: Springer, 2018), https://doi.org/10.1007/978-3-319-89866-7_5.
9. Emilie C. Rijnink et al., "Tissue Microchimerism Is Increased during Pregnancy: A Human Autopsy Study," *Molecular Human Reproduction,* Volume 21.11 (November 2015), 857–64, https://doi.org/10.1093/molehr/gav047.
10. Suzanne E Peterson et al., "Fetal Cellular Microchimerism in Miscarriage and Pregnancy Termination," *Chimerism* 4.4 (May 3, 2013): 136–38, https://doi.org/10.4161/chim.24915.
11. Ibid.
12. "ACOG Committee Opinion No. 385: The Limits of Conscientious Refusal in Reproductive Medicine," *Obstetrics & Gynecology* 110, no. 5 (November 2007): 1203–1208, https://doi.org/10.1097/01.aog.0000291561.48203.27; available at https://www.acog.org/en/Clinical/Clinical%20Guidance/Committee%20Opinion/Articles/2007/11/The%20Limits%20of%20Conscientious%20Refusal%20in%20Reproductive%20Medicine.
13. Kathleen M. Roe, "Private Troubles and Public Issues: Providing Abortion amid Competing Definitions," *Social Science & Medicine,* Volume 29.10 (1989), 1191–98, https://www.sciencedirect.com/science/article/abs/pii/0277953689903626.
14. Rachel M. MacNair, "The Nightmares of Choice: The Psychological Effects of Performing Abortions," *Touchstone* (The Fellowship of St. James, September 2003), https://www.touchstonemag.com/archives/article.php?id=16-07-022-f.
15. Marla J. Marek, "Nurses' Attitudes Toward Pregnancy Termination in the Labor and Delivery Setting," *Journal of Obstetric, Gynecologic & Neonatal Nursing* 33.4 (July 1, 2004): 472–79, https://doi.org/10.1177/0884217504266912.
16. William F. May, *The Physician's Covenant: Images of the Healer in Medical Ethics,* 2nd ed. (Louisville: Westminster John Knox, 2000), 47.
17. Ibid.
18. Ibid., ch. 4.
19. Edmund D. Pellegrino and David C. Thomasma, *The Virtues in Medical Practice* (Oxford: Oxford University Press, 1993), 69.
20. Ibid, 76.

21. A. T. Robertson, *Word Pictures of the New Testament* (Louisville: B&H, 1933), biblestudytools.com, https://www.biblestudytools.com/commentaries/robertsons-word-pictures/matthew/matthew-5-18.html.
22. M. G. Easton, "Tittle," in *Illustrated Bible Dictionary*, 3rd ed. (New York: Thomas Nelson, 1897), biblestudytools.com, https://www.biblestudytools.com/dictionary/tittle/.
23. William G. T. Shedd, "Introductory Essay," in *Nicene and Post-Nicene Fathers*, ed. Philip Schaff (Buffalo, NY: Christian Literature Co., 1887), series 1, vol. 3 https://ccel.org/ccel/schaff/npnf103/npnf103.iv.i.i.html.
24. Thomas Aquinas, *The Summa Theologica* (Cincinnati, OH: Benzinger, 1947), I.93.2, https://www.ccel.org/ccel/aquinas/summa/FP/FP093.html.
25. Anthony Hoekema, *Created in God's Image* (Grand Rapids: Eerdmans, 1986), 13.
26. Millard J. Erickson, *Christian Theology*, 3rd ed. (Grand Rapids: Baker Academic, 2013), 436.
27. Jane Doe, "There Just Wasn't Room."
28. F. W. Boreham, "'The Sword of Solomon,'" in *The Blue Flame*, reprint ed. (Pioneer Library, 2018 [1930]), 23–36.
29. Ibid., 29.
30. Ibid., 32–33.
31. David M. Fergusson, L. John Horwood, and Joseph M. Boden, "Abortion and Mental Health Disorders: Evidence from a 30-Year Longitudinal Study," *British Journal of Psychiatry* 193.6 (2008): 444–51, https://doi.org/10.1192/bjp.bp.108.056499.
32. All Bible translations for the remainder of the chapter are from the New International Version (NIV).

Chapter 8: Marvelously Revealed: The Symphony of a Woman's Body

1. There are two drugs now on the market that block the action of progesterone in a woman's body. One of these drugs is Mifeprex, also known as mifepristone. This drug was FDA-approved to be used to cause abortions. The other drug is Ella. This drug was approved as a "morning after pill contraceptive," to be taken in the second half of the cycle to "prevent pregnancy." They are both the same type of drug, called *progesterone blockers* (for a full discussion, see AAPLOG Medical Management of Elective Induced Abortion [https://aaplog.org/wp-content/uploads/2020/03/FINAL-PB-8-Medical-Management-of-Elective-Induced-Abortion.pdf]). Both drugs block progesterone from causing the changes in a woman's womb that would allow her body to nourish and feed her preborn child. If her embryo has not yet implanted, both of these drugs interrupt the preparation of the womb, which allows the baby to implant. If her embryo has implanted and is growing, both of these drugs can cause the lining of the womb to disintegrate, starving the preborn child until it dies.

   There is one very, very important thing to note, however. If a woman takes the abortion drug Mifeprex and she changes her mind about the abortion, the progesterone-blocking effects of Mifeprex may be overcome if she takes large doses of progesterone to counteract the effects of the progesterone blockade. There is evidence that taking progesterone quickly, within 72 hours of taking mifepristone, increases the chances that the baby will survive, from about 25 percent to about 68 percent. It is not perfect. But taking "progesterone rescue" gives the baby a second chance at life.

2. Maureen L. Condic, "When Does Human Life Begin? A Scientific Perspective," Westchester Institute White Paper 1.1 (October 2008): 1–18, Westchester Institute for Ethics & the Human Person, Thornwood, NY, https://bdfund.org/wp-content/uploads/2016/05/wi_whitepaper_life_print.pdf. This paper was later published with the same title in the *National Catholic Bioethics Quarterly* 9.1 (2009): 12949, https://doi.org/10.5840/ncbq20099184. See also idem, "When Does Human Life Begin? The Scientific Evidence and Terminology Revisited," *University of St. Thomas Journal of Law and Public Policy* 8, no. 1 (Fall 2013): 44–81, http://www.embryodefense.org/MaureenCondicSET.pdf.
3. Maureen A. Knippen, "Microchimerism: Sharing Genes in Illness and in Health," *ISRN Nursing* (May 2011): 1–4, https://doi.org/10.5402/2011/893819. Suzanne E. Peterson et al., "Fetal Cellular Microchimerism in Miscarriage and Pregnancy Termination," *Chimerism* 4, no. 4 (October 1, 2013): 136–38, https://www.ncbi.nlm.nih.gov/pmc/articles/PMC3921195/.
4. For a full discussion, see American Association of Pro-Life Obstetricians and Gynecologists (AAPLOG) Abortion and Breast Cancer Committee Opinion 8, https://aaplog.org/wp-content/uploads/2020/01/FINAL-CO-8-Abortion-Breast-Cancer-1.9.20.pdf.
5. For a full discussion, see ibid.
6. For a full discussion, see AAPLOG Abortion and Preterm Birth, https://aaplog.org/wp-content/uploads/2019/12/FINAL-PRACTICE-BULLETIN-5-Abortion-Preterm-Birth.pdf.
7. For a full discussion, see AAPLOG Abortion and Mental Health, https://aaplog.org/wp-content/uploads/2019/12/FINAL-Abortion-Mental-Health-PB7.pdf.
8. See, e.g., https://www.focusonthefamily.ca/content/post-abortion-healing; https://www.usccb.org/prolife/abortion-healing; https://www.heartbeatservices.org/abortion-recovery; https://sistersoflife.org/healing-after-abortion/; https://www.care-net.org/i-had-an-abortion.

Chapter 9: The Myth of the Unwanted Child: How Adoption Powerfully Dispels the Lie

1. Margaret Sanger, *Women and the New Race* (New York: Truth Publishing, 1920), 229, https://www.bartleby.com/1013/18.html (paragraph 8).
2. Ibid., 74, https://www.bartleby.com/1013/6.html (paragraph 5).
3. https://www.charitynavigator.org/ein/231352509.
4. https://www.influencewatach.org/app/uploads/2019/10/PPFA-Margaret-Sanger-Fact-Sheet-10.2019.
5. TheRadianceFoundation.org.

6. https://www.acf.hhs.gov/sites/default/files/documents/cb/afcarsreport27.pdf.
7. Joe Carter, "FactChecker: Could U.S. Churches Solve the Orphan Crisis?," The Gospel Coalition, May 28, 2019, https://www.thegospelcoalition.org/article/factchecker-u-s-churches-solve-orphan-crisis/.
8. Ibid.

Chapter 10: Mom, Thank You for Choosing Life: The Perspective of an Abortion Survivor

1. For the *New York Times* report on Dr. Kermit Gosnell's conviction, see https://nyti.ms/ZVrwMU. Cf. Court of Common Pleas, First Judicial District of Pennsylvania Criminal Justice Division, Grand Jury Report, https://cdn.cnsnews.com/documents/Gosnell,%20Grand%20Jury%20Report.pdf.
2. *June Medical Services v. Russo*, Amicus Curiae Americans United for Life, https://www.supremecourt.gov/DocketPDF/18/18-1460/103796/20190624094927367_18-1460%20Amicus%20Brief%20of%20Americans%20United%20for%20Life.pdf (pages 25–26).
3. Court of Appeal of Louisiana, Fourth Circuit. *Meranda Varnardo v. Gentilly Medical Clinic for Women.*
4. C. H. Spurgeon, *The Treasury of David*, vol. 6 (New York: Funk and Wagnalls, 1882), 285.
5. https://www.guttmacher.org/news-release/2017/abortion-common-experience-us-women-despite-dramatic-declines-rates.
6. Christine Dehlendorf et al., "Disparities in Abortion Rates: A Public Health Approach," *American Journal of Public Health* 103 (2013): 1772–79, https://www.ncbi.nlm.nih.gov/pmc/articles/PMC3780732/.
7. Ibid. Cf. James Studnicki, John W. Fisher, and James L. Sherley, "Perceiving and Addressing the Pervasive Racial Disparity in Abortion," *Health Services Research and Managerial Epidemiology* 7 (2020), https://doi.org/10.1177/2333392820949743.
8. Tara C. Jatlaoui et al., "Abortion Surveillance—United States, 2015," Centers for Disease Control and Prevention, Mortality and Morbidity Weekly Report (MMWR), *Surveillance Summaries* 67, no. 13 (2018): 1–45, https://www.cdc.gov/mmwr/volumes/67/ss/ss6713a1.htm.
9. Gillian Aston and Susan Bewley, "Abortion and Domestic Violence," *The Obstetrician & Gynecologist* 11 (2009): 163–68, https://www.researchgate.net/publication/250980683_Abortion_and_domestic_violence.

Chapter 11: Embracing Life's Bump: Experiencing God's Grace in Teenage Pregnancy

1. Amy Ford, *A Bump in Life: True Stories of Hope and Courage during an Unplanned Pregnancy* (Hurst, TX: Embrace Grace, 2018).
2. "U.S. Teen Pregnancy, Birth and Abortion Rates Reach the Lowest Levels in Almost Four Decades," Guttmacher Institute, April 5, 2016, https://www

.guttmacher.org/news-release/2016/us-teen-pregnancy-birth-and-abortion-rates-reach-lowest-levels-almost-four-decades.

3. Anne Dellinger, *Public School and Pregnant and Parenting Adolescents: A Legal Guide* (School of Government, University of North Carolina: Chapel Hill, 2004), https://www.sog.unc.edu/sites/www.sog.unc.edu/files/full_text_books/PubSchool_PregAd_final.pdf.
4. Grace Chen, "Pregnant in Public School: Challenges and Options," Public School Review, February 10, 2020, https://www.publicschoolreview.com/blog/pregnant-in-public-school-challenges-and-options.
5. "Get Help Paying for Child Care," ChildCare.gov, https://childcare.gov/consumer-education/get-help-paying-for-child-care.
6. "Kids on Campus: Colleges Offering Child Care," Accredited Schools Online, December 7, 2020, https://www.accreditedschoolsonline.org/resources/colleges-offering-child-care/.
7. Sarah's story is told in Amy Ford, *A Bump in Life*, 111–17.

Chapter 12: Hope Is Found in Hard Places: Pregnant during Financial Hardship

1. See https://www.youtube.com/watch?v=I6XfU8KVkzI, or the film's official website, https://www.maafa21.com.

Chapter 13: But God Intended It for Good—Finding Purpose in Pregnancy from Rape

1. A few days after the rape, I went to my OB-GYN to be examined, to check for STDs, and so on. The police department in my area had come under scrutiny for not testing rape kits. I knew this because of extensive research I had done in college that I actually presented to the city government. I was far too familiar with the lack of care shown by the police to want to go through the extremely intense process of having a rape kit done after being violated, knowing it wouldn't make much of a difference. I encourage every woman to make her own decision about whether or not to report a rape.
2. http://www.HopeAfterRapeConception.org/.
3. Amy Sobie and David C. Reardon, "A Survey of Rape and Incest Pregnancies," in *Victims and Victors: Speaking Out About Their Pregnancies, Abortions, and Children Resulting from Sexual Assault*, eds. D. C. Reardon, J. Makimaa, and A. Sobie (Springfield, IL: Acorn, 2000), 18–24, at 19.

Chapter 14: Fearfully and Wonderfully Made: Reimagining Pregnancy When the Baby Has Disabilities

1. Melissa Conrad Stöppler, "Quad Marker Screening Test Uses, Accuracy, Results, and False Positive," MedicineNet, https://www.medicinenet.com/quad_marker_screen_test/article.htm#what_should_you_do_if_you_have_normal_or_abnormal_tests_results.

2. The United States Holocaust Memorial Museum: "The Murder of the Handicapped," Holocaust Encyclopedia, https://encyclopedia.ushmm.org/content/en/article/the-murder-of-the-handicapped.
3. Randy Alcorn, *Pro-Life Answers to Pro-Choice Arguments* (New York: Crown Publishing, 2009), 228. Cf. J. Lloyd and K. Laurence, "Response to Termination of Pregnancy for Genetic Reasons," *Zeitschrift für Kinderchirurgie* 38, suppl. 2 (1983): 98–99; B. Blumberg et al., "The Psychological Sequelae of Abortion Performed for Genetic Indication," *American Journal of Obstetrics and Gynecology* 2 (1975): 215–24.

Chapter 15: Are Abortions Ever Medically Necessary? A Life-Affirming Approach to Complex Pregnancies

1. For the RHA, see https://legislation.nysenate.gov/pdf/bills/2019/S240.
2. "FAQs about the Reproductive Health Act," The New York Senate (February 12, 2019). https://www.nysenate.gov/newsroom/articles/2019/liz-krueger/faqs-about-reproductive-health-act, emphasis added.
3. https://www.prochoiceamerica.org/state-law/new-york/, emphasis added.
4. Diana Greene Foster and Katrina Kimport, "Who Seeks Abortions at or After 20 Weeks?" *Perspectives on Sexual and Reproductive Health* 45.4 (2013): 2010–18, https://www.guttmacher.org/journals/psrh/2013/11/who-seeks-abortions-or-after-20-weeks.
5. James Studnicki, "Late-Term Abortion and Medical Necessity: A Failure of Science," *Health Services Research and Managerial Epidemiology* 6 (2019), https://www.ncbi.nlm.nih.gov/pmc/articles/PMC6457018/.
6. "Fact Checking the Fact Checkers: Abortionists Misrepresent the Facts," AAPLOG, https://aaplog.org/fact-checking-the-fact-checkers-abortionists-misrepresent-the-facts/.
7. Donald Weber, "Be Aware of Risk Factors, Signs of Premature Birth," Mayo Clinic Health System, https://www.mayoclinichealthsystem.org/hometown-health/speaking-of-health/be-aware-of-risk-factors-signs-of-premature-birth.
8. https://aaplog.org/wp-content/uploads/2019/12/FINAL-Policy-Statement-Fact-Sheet-Fetal-Pain.pdf.
9. Susan L. Hasegawa and Jessica T. Fry, "Moving Toward a Shared Process: The Impact of Parent Experiences on Perinatal Palliative Care," *Seminars in Perinatology* 41 (2017): 95–100, https://doi.org/10.1053/j.semperi.2016.11.002.
10. Dan Grossman and Robyn Shickler, "Lila Rose claim that 'abortion is never medically necessary' is inaccurate; it is necessary in certain cases to preserve mother's life," Science Feedback (August 30, 2019), https://sciencefeedback.co/claimreview/lila-rose-claim-that-abortion-is-never-medically-necessary-is-inaccurate-it-is-necessary-in-certain-cases-to-preserve-mothers-life-young-america-foundation/.
11. "Fact checking the Fact checkers: Abortionists misrepresent the facts," AAPLOG, https://aaplog.org/fact-checking-the-fact-checkers-abortionists-misrepresent-the-facts/.

12. https://www.dublindeclaration.com/.
13. "Former Abortionist: Dr. David Brewer," Life Institute, https://thelifeinstitute.net/learning-centre/abortion-facts/providers/former-abortionists/dr-david-brewer.

Chapter 16: The Truth about Post-Abortive Trauma: The Personal Account of a Survivor and Activist

1. As Angela Lanfranchi, Ian Gentles, and Elizabeth Ring-Cassidy lament, "Because of the highly controversial nature of the mental health consequences of abortion, it is extremely difficult to carry out objective, scientific research in this area. Abortion's impact on women's mental health is simply too politically charged an issue. As in other areas, such as climate change or nutrition, once a politically correct position has been established, any publications that challenge that position tend to be ignored, dismissed or undermined" ("Depression, Suicide, Substance Abuse: Contested Research," in *Complications: Abortion's Impact on Women*, 2nd ed. [Toronto: deVeber Institute for Bioethics and Social Research, 2018], 277–89, at 277). These authors also acknowledge that many post-abortive women are overlooked in the research: "Post-abortion studies can never accurately measure the experiences of many women. Many of those who struggle with mental health problems following an abortion are not represented in the statistic studies of abortion and yet these women exist. We know about them through their stories, their affidavits and their testimonies" (289).
2. See Lanfranchi, Gentles, and Ring-Cassidy, *Complications*, 91–258.
3. See the meta-analysis of Priscilla K. Coleman, who showed that "women who had undergone an abortion experienced an 81% increased risk of mental health problems, and nearly 10% of the incidence of mental health problems was shown to be attributable to abortion" ("Abortion and Mental Health: Quantitative Synthesis and Analysis of Research Published 1995–2009," *British Journal of Psychiatry* 199.3 [2011]: 180–86), https://www.cambridge.org/core/journals/the-british-journal-of-psychiatry/article/abortion-and-mental-health-quantitative-synthesis-and-analysis-of-research-published-19952009/E8D556AAE1C1D2F0F8B060B28BEE6C3D.
4. The scientific research shows much the same: "The testimonies of post-abortive women reveal their psychological pain in a variety of ways: a woman may become depressed or anxious; . . . she may also engage in harmful behaviours in an attempt to suppress the pain. Regardless of its expression, the psychological pain associated with elective abortion is inextricably linked with guilt" (Lanfranchi, Gentles, and Ring-Cassidy, "Depression, Suicide, Substance Abuse," 289).
5. For additional testimonies, see Angela Lanfranchi, Ian Gentles, and Elizabeth Ring-Cassidy, "Who Are the Experts? What 101 Women Told Us," and "Women's Voices: Narratives of the Abortion Experience," in *Complications*, 309–24 and 325–62 respectively.
6. Guy Condon and David Hazard, similarly, list the following as "aftershocks of male postabortion trauma": difficulty with commitment, dodging authority, no

solid sense of identity, working to impress moral leaders, keeping women at bay, trouble bonding, fearing impending tragedy, failing to own mistakes, feeling inadequate as a leader (*Fatherhood Aborted: The Profound Effects of Abortion on Men* [Carol Stream, IL: Tyndale House Publishers, 2001], 2–9).

Chapter 17: An Expedient Tool: The Harmful Effects of Abortion on Society

1. "Aspiration Abortion: First Trimester Suction D&C," Abortion Procedures: What You Need to Know, https://www.abortionprocedures.com/aspiration/.
2. "D&E," Abortion Procedures: What You Need to Know, https://www.abortionprocedures.com/; Patrina Mosley, "Dismemberment Abortion," Family Research Council, June 2018, https://downloads.frc.org/EF/EF18F25.pdf.
3. Patrina Mosley, "Why We Need the Born-Alive Abortion Survivors Protection Act," Townhall, February 25, 2020, https://townhall.com/columnists/patrinamosley/2020/02/25/why-we-need-the-bornalive-abortion-survivors-protection-act-n2561807.
4. Calvin Freiburger, "Michigan Gov. Whitmer says abortions must continue because they're 'life-sustaining,'" LifeSite News, April 17, 2020, https://www.lifesitenews.com/news/michigan-gov-whitmer-says-abortions-must-continue-because-theyre-life-sustaining.
5. Elective abortion are abortions that are not carried out for medical purposes such as for the life of the mother, but simply carried out by request of the mother. The overwhelming majority of abortions performed in the United States are elective.
6. "Practice Bulletin—Abortion and Mental Health," American Association of Pro-life Obstetricians & Gynecologists, December 30, 2019, https://aaplog.org/wp-content/uploads/2019/12/FINAL-Abortion-Mental-Health-PB7.pdf.
7. "Induced Abortion in the United States," Guttmacher Institute, September 2019, https://www.guttmacher.org/fact-sheet/induced-abortion-united-states; "Study of Women who have had an Abortion and Their Views on Church," LifeWay Research, 2015, https://lifewayresearch.com/wp-content/uploads/2015/11/Care-Net-Final-Presentation-Report-Revised.pdf.
8. David C. Reardon, "The Abortion and Mental Health Controversy: A Comprehensive Literature Review of Common Ground Agreements, Disagreements, Actionable Recommendations, and Research Opportunities," *SAGE Open Medicine* 6 (2018): 1–38, https://www.ncbi.nlm.nih.gov/pmc/articles/PMC6207970/.
9. Tara C. Jatlaoui et al., "Abortion Surveillance—United States, 2016," Centers for Disease Control and Prevention, Mortality and Morbidity Weekly Report (MMWR), *Surveillance Summaries* 68.11 (2019): 1–41, https://www.cdc.gov/mmwr/volumes/68/ss/ss6811a1.htm?s_cid=ss6811a1_w.
10. "U.S. Abortion Statistics," Abort73.com, January 21, 2020, https://abort73.com/abortion_facts/us_abortion_statistics/.
11. Lawrence B. Finer et al., "Reasons U.S. Women Have Abortions: Quantitative and Qualitative Perspectives," *Perspectives on Sexual and Reproductive Health* 37.3

(2005): 110–18, https://www.guttmacher.org/sites/default/files/article_files/3711005.pdf.

12. "Intimate Partner Violence," American College of Obstetricians and Gynecologists: *Committee Opinion*, No. 518 (2012), https://www.acog.org/clinical/clinical-guidance/committee-opinion/articles/2012/02/intimate-partner-violence.
13. Laura J. Lederer and Christopher A. Wetzel, "The Health Consequences of Sex Trafficking and Their Implications for Identifying Victims in Healthcare Facilities," *Beazley Institute for Health Law and Policy* 23.1 (2014): 61–91, https://www.globalcenturion.org/wp-content/uploads/2014/08/The-Health-Consequences-of-Sex-Trafficking.pdf.
14. Catherine T. Coyle and Vincent M. Rue, "Men's Perceptions Concerning Disclosure of a Partner's Abortion: Implications for Counseling," *The European Journal of Counseling Psychology* 3.2 (2015) (https://ejcop.psychopen.eu/article/view/54/html); idem, "Men's Experience of Elective Abortion: A Mixed Methods Study of Loss," *Journal of Pastoral Counseling* 45 (2010): 4–31, https://www.menandabortion.net/wp-content/uploads/2015/07/NOV_Coyle_Rue_2010.pdf.
15. Thomas R. Malthus, *An Essay on the Principle of Population* (London: J. Johnson, 1798), http://www.esp.org/books/malthus/population/malthus.pdf.
16. Charles Darwin, *On the Origin of Species by Means of Natural Selection, or the Preservation of Favoured Races in the Struggle for Life* (London: J. Murray, 1859), https://www.loc.gov/resource/rbctos.2017gen17473?r=-0.742,-0.085,2.485,1.579,0.
17. Francis Galton, "Chapter XXI. Race Improvement," in *Memories of My Life* (London: Methuen & Co, 1908), http://galton.org/books/memories/chapter-XXI.html.
18. Denis R. Alexander and Ronald L. Numbers, eds. *Biology and Ideology from Descartes to Dawkins* (Chicago: University of Chicago Press: 2010), 169.
19. Margaret Sanger, *Pivot of Civilization* (New York: Brentano's, 1922), 181, http://www.gutenberg.org/files/1689/1689-h/1689-h.htm#link2H_4_0017.
20. Margaret Sanger, Personal Letter to Clarence Gamble, December 10, 1939, *Sophia Smith Collection*: Women's History Archives, Smith College, https://libex.smith.edu/omeka/files/original/d6358bc3053c93183295bf2df1c0c931.pdf.
21. "Abortion Surveillance—United States, 2016," Centers for Disease Control and Prevention, *Mortality and Morbidity Weekly Report (MMWR).*
22. Sonya Rastogi et al., "The Black Population: 2010," United States Census Bureau, September 2011, http://www.census.gov/prod/cen2010/briefs/c2010br-06.pdf.
23. "Frederick Osborn, Galton and Mid-Century Eugenics, 1956 Eugenics Review published lecture and 'Voluntary Unconscious Selection,'" Eugenics and Other Evils, accessed June 25, 2020, http://eugenics.us/frederick-osborn-galton-and-mid-century-eugenics-1956-eugenics-review-published-lecture-and-voluntary-unconscious-selection/247.htm.

24. Sanger, *Pivot of Civilization*, 183.
25. Patrina Mosley, "Why the Hysteria Over *Roe*? Because It Would Strike a Blow to Eugenics," Family Research Council, July 6, 2018, https://www.frcblog.com/2018/07/why-hysteria-over-emroeem-because-it-would-strike-blow-eugenics/; https://supreme.justia.com/cases/federal/us/410/113/#T62.
26. *Roe v. Wade*, 410 U.S. 113 (1973), https://www.law.cornell.edu/supremecourt/text/410/113.
27. *Buck v. Bell*, 274 U.S. 200 (1927), https://supreme.justia.com/cases/federal/us/274/200/.
28. Emily Bazelon, "The Place of Women on the Court," *The New York Times Magazine*, July 7, 2009, https://www.nytimes.com/2009/07/12/magazine/12ginsburg-t.html.
29. "Pro-Abortion Letter from Lawyer Ron Weddington to President-Elect Bill Clinton," Scribd, https://www.scribd.com/document/252535824/Pro-abortion-letter-from-Lawyer-Ron-Weddington-to-President-elect-Bill-Clinton; https://www.afterabortion.org/PAR/V14/RU486letter.htm.
30. Katy Grimes, "Gov. Newsom Signs Bill Mandating Free Abortions at All Colleges and Universities," California Globe, October 12, 2019, https://californiaglobe.com/section-2/gov-newsom-signs-bill-mandating-free-abortions-at-all-colleges-and-universities/.
31. "Order List: 587 U.S.," U.S. Supreme Court, May 28, 2019, https://www.supremecourt.gov/orders/courtorders/052819zor_2dq3.pdf.
32. Julian Quinones and Arijeta Lajka, "'What kind of society do you want to live in?': Inside the country where Down syndrome is disappearing," CBS News, August 14, 2017, https://www.cbsnews.com/news/down-syndrome-iceland/.
33. "The Effects of China's One-Child Policy," *Encyclopedia Britannica*, https://www.britannica.com/story/the-effects-of-chinas-one-child-policy; Quanbao Jiang, "Gender imbalance and the marriage squeeze in China," The Asia Dialogue, November 18, 2019, https://theasiadialogue.com/2019/11/18/gender-imbalance-and-the-marriage-squeeze-in-china/.
34. Arthur Erken, *State of World Population 2020*, United Nations Population Fund, https://www.unfpa.org/sites/default/files/pub-pdf/UNFPA_PUB_2020_EN_State_of_World_Population.pdf.
35. Amanda Stirone Mansfield, "Overview of Legislation and Litigation Involving Protections Against Down Syndrome Discrimination Abortion," Charlotte Lozier Institute, March 21, 2019, https://lozierinstitute.org/overview-legislation-litigation-involving-protections-against-down-syndrome-discrimination-abortion/.
36. Patrina Mosley, "Justice Thomas: The Roots of Abortion Are Eugenics," Family Research Council, May 28, 2019, https://www.frcblog.com/2019/05/justice-thomas-roots-abortion-are-eugenics/.
37. U.S. Agency for International Development, "Acting Administrator John Barsa Letter to UN Secretary General Guterres," press release, May 18, 2020, https://

www.usaid.gov/news-information/press-releases/may-18-2020-acting-administrator-john-barsa-un-secretary-general-antonio-guterres.

38. Patrina Mosley, "USAID Tells UN That Abortion Is Not 'Humanitarian Aid'," Family Research Council, May 20, 2020, https://www.frcblog.com/2020/05/usaid-tells-un-abortion-not-humanitarian-aid/; Tony Perkins, "Family Research Council Praises Trump Administration for Expanding Pro-Life Mexico City Policy," press release, March 26, 2019, https://www.frc.org/get.cfm?i=PR19C03.
39. "We Believe," Bill and Melinda Gates Foundation, https://www.gatesfoundation.org/.
40. Mairead McArdle, "Sanders Knocked for Comments Linking Abortion to Population Control," *National Review*, September 5, 2019, https://www.nationalreview.com/news/sanders-knocked-for-comments-linking-abortion-to-population-control/; Chelsea Follett, "Politicians' Support for Population Control Is Dangerous," CATO Institute, September 13, 2019, https://www.cato.org/publications/commentary/politicians-support-population-control-dangerous.
41. Al Gore, *Earth in the Balance* (Boston: Houghton Mifflin, 1992), 307.
42. "China Allows Three Children in Major Policy Shift," May 31, 2021, https://www.bbc.com/news/world-asia-china-57303592.
43. Patrina Mosley, "Why the Hysteria Over *Roe*; "Frederick Osborn: 'birth control and abortion are turning out to be great eugenic advances,'" Eugenics and Other Evils, http://eugenics.us/frederick-osborn-birth-control-and-abortion-are-turning-out-to-be-great-eugenic-advances/256.htm.

Chapter 18: The Voices and Values of the New Pro-Life Generation

1. "10 Years of the MILLENNIAL Impact Report, Case Foundation, July 26, 2019, casefoundation.org/resource/10-years-of-the-millennial-impact/report. July 2019, casefoundation.org/program/millennial-engagement/.
2. "Social Justice," Merriam-Webster, www.merriam-webster.com/dictionary/social justice.
3. Leslie J. Reagan, *When Abortion Was a Crime: Women, Medicine, and Law in the United States, 1867–1973* (Berkley: University of California Press, 2008).
4. "Annual Report 2011-2012," Planned Parenthood, https://www.plannedparenthood.org/files/4913/9620/1413/PPFA_AR_2012_121812_vF.pdf.
5. "2014–2015 Annual Report," Planned Parenthood, https://www.plannedparenthood.org/uploads/filer_public/71/63/71633f42-af81-43e2-90c3-2e5fff989c91/2014-2015_ppfa_annual_report_.pdf.
6. "2017–2018 Annual Report," Planned Parenthood https://www.plannedparenthood.org/uploads/filer_public/80/d7/80d7d7c7-977c-4036-9c61-b3801741b441/190118-annualreport18-p01.pdf.
7. "Annual Report 2018–2019," Planned Parenthood, https://www.plannedparenthood.org/uploads/filer_public/2e/da/2eda3f50-82aa-4ddb-acce-c2854c4ea80b/2018-2019_annual_report.pdf.

8. Melanie Israel, "Planned Parenthood Sets New Record for Abortions in a Single Year" The Heritage Foundation, Jan. 9, 2020, www.heritage.org/life/commentary/planned-parenthood-sets-new-record-abortions-single-year.
9. "Medication Abortion," Guttmacher Institute, Nov. 21, 2019, www.guttmacher.org/evidence-you-can-use/medication-abortion.
10. Watch the new docuseries *This Is Chemical Abortion,* www.thisischemicalabortion.com/video/series/. Charlotte has contributed to and created pro-life projects including in conjunction with Students for Life of America and Heartbeat International. She recently created the above-mentioned project addressing the dangers of the abortion pill.
11. Shout Your Abortion, www.shoutyourabortion.com/.
12. "Abortion Healing," USCCB, www.usccb.org/prolife/abortion-healing.
13. Emma Green, "When Your Pregnancy Is Political," *The Atlantic,* July 8, 2019, www.theatlantic.com/politics/archive/2019/07/lila-rose-anti-abortion/593404/.
14. Maria Dinzeo, "Jury Finds Abortion Foes Harmed Planned Parenthood, Awards Over $2 Million," Courthouse News Service, Nov. 16, 2019, www.courthousenews.com/jury-finds-abortion-foes-harmed-planned-parenthood-awards-870k/.
15. Jennifer Gerson Uffalussy, "State Probes Find Zero Planned Parenthood Violations as Antiabortion Group Is Sued Over Undercover Videos," July 13, 2015, Yahoo!, https://www.yahoo.com/lifestyle/state-probes-find-zero-planned-parenthood-125533982837.html.
16. "David Daleiden Indicted on Felony Charge by Texas Grand Jury," Planned Parenthood, www.plannedparenthood.org/about-us/newsroom/press-releases/david-daleiden-indicted-on-felony-charge-by-texas-grand-jury?gclid=Cj0KCQjwtsv7BRCmARIsANu-CQeEvvU4HUafBOLzftS8lUohQ-Kaz2fXWtwNDiVy2ivF9owJjX7UHpsIaAmd8EALw_wcB.
17. Staff, SFLA Action, "Students for Life Action Calls on Pro-Life Legislators Nationwide to Implement The Pro-Life Generation's Blueprint for a Post-Roe America," SFLA Action, August 24, 2020, studentsforlifeaction.org/students-for-life-action-calls-on-pro-life-legislators-nationwide-to-implement-the-pro-life-generations-blueprint-for-a-post-roe-america/.

Charlotte has connections with Live Action and will be attending Live Action's gala this year at the expense of the organization as a guest.

Chapter 19: The Hands and Feet of Jesus: How Pregnancy Centers Care for Women and Men

1. Client advocates are trained pregnancy center personnel who are equipped to come alongside clients and provide assistance in exploring their pregnancy options, screening for adverse situations, and providing referrals to needed community resources.
2. According to the WHO's International Forum for Social Development, social justice is a relatively new concept that addresses six primary inequalities among

people groups: (1) Inequalities in the distribution of income; (2) Inequalities in the distribution of assets; (3) Inequalities in the distribution of opportunities for work and remunerated employment; (4) Inequalities in the distribution of access to knowledge; (5) Inequalities in the distribution of health services, social security and the provision of a safe environment; (6) Inequalities in the distribution of opportunities for civic and political participation.

3. Timothy Keller, *Generous Justice: How God's Grace Makes Us Just* (New York: Riverhead Books, 2010), 18.
4. "Induced Abortion in the United States: September 2019 Fact Sheet," Guttmacher Institute, https://www.guttmacher.org/fact-sheet/induced-abortion-united-states.
5. *Pregnancy Centers Stand the Test of Time*, A Legacy of Life and Love Report Series (Arlington, VA: Charlotte Lozier Institute, 2020), 16, https://lozierinstitute.org/wp-content/uploads/2020/10/Pregnancy-Center-Report-2020_FINAL.pdf.
6. "Sexually Transmitted Diseases: Adolescents and Young Adults," Centers for Disease Control and Prevention, https://www.cdc.gov/std/life-stages-populations/adolescents-youngadults.htm.
7. *Pregnancy Centers Stand the Test of Time*, 17–18; "Adolescents and Young Adults," Centers for Disease Control and Prevent, https://www.cdc.gov/std/life-stages-populations/adolescents-youngadults.htm.
8. In 2019, 5 percent of centers provided some level of prenatal care, while 2 percent offered pap tests and well woman visits (*Pregnancy Centers Stand the Test of Time*, 18).
9. Ibid., 16.
10. Ibid.
11. J. S. Shah et al. "Improving Rates of Early Entry Prenatal Care in an Underserved Population," *Maternal and Child Health Journal* 22.12 (2018): 1738–42 (doi:10.1007/s10995-018-2569-z).
12. *Pregnancy Centers Stand the Test of Time*, 16.
13. P. K. Coleman et al., "Predictors and Correlates of Abortion in the Fragile Families and Well-Being Study: Paternal Behavior, Substance Use, and Partner Violence," *International Journal of Mental Health and Addiction*, 7.3 (2009): 405–22, https://link.springer.com/article/10.1007%2Fs11469-008-9188-7.
14. M. Öberg, "Prevalence of Intimate Partner Violence among Women Seeking Termination of Pregnancy Compared to Women Seeking Contraceptive Counseling," *Acta Obsetetricia et Gynecologica Scandinavica*, 93.1 (2014): 45–51, doi:10.1111/aogs.12279; C. C. Pallitto et al., "Intimate Partner Violence, Abortion, and Unintended Pregnancy: Results from the WHO Multi-Country Study on Women's Health and Domestic Violence," *International Journal of Gynecology and Obstetrics* 120.1 (2013): 3–9, https://doi.org/10.1016/j.ijgo.2012.07.003; K. S. Chibber et al., "The Role of Intimate Partners in Women's Reasons for Seeking Abortion," *Women's Health Issues* 24.1 (2014): 131–38, doi:10.1016/j.whi.2013.10.007.

15. Becky Yeh, "Planned Parenthood Lied to the Media about Retraining Thousands of Staff How to Report Child Sex Trafficking," Live Action, January 17, 2017, https://www.liveaction.org/news/planned-parenthood-lied-media-retraining-thousands-staff-report-child-sex-trafficking/.
16. See *Planned Parenthood v. Danforth*, 428 U.S. 52 (1976).
17. D. M. Fergusson, L. J. Horwood, and J. M. Boden, "Abortion and Mental Health Disorders: Evidence from a 30-Year Longitudinal Study," *British Journal of Psychiatry* 193 (2008): 444–51, http://bjp.rcpsych.org/content/193/6/444.full; P. S. Shah and J. Zao, "Induced Termination of Pregnancy and Low Birthweight and Preterm Birth: A Systematic Review and Meta-Analyses," British Journal of Obstetrics & Gynaecology 116.11 (2009): 1425–42, doi: 10.1111/j.1471-0528.2009.02278.x; D. C. Reardon, P. K. Coleman, and J. Cougle, "Substance Use Associated with Prior History of Abortion and Unintended Birth: A National Cross Sectional Cohort Study," *American Journal of Drug and Alcohol Abuse* 26 (2004): 369–83; Y. Huang et al., "A Meta-Analysis of the Association between Induced Abortion and Breast Cancer Risk among Chinese Females," *Cancer Causes & Control* 25.2 (2014): 227–36, http://link.springer.com/article/10.1007/s10552-013-0325-7.
18. In 2019, centers provided nearly one million free consultations with an estimated value of $28 million (*Pregnancy Centers Stand the Test of Time*, 16).
19. Affiliation organizations such as Care Net, NIFLA, and Heartbeat International.
20. See, e.g., Silent No More Awareness, http://silentnomoreawareness.org/testimonies/testimony.aspx?ID=3128.
21. Linda Cochrane, *Forgiven and Set Free* (Grand Rapids: Baker, 2015).
22. Care Net's vision statement reads: "Care Net envisions a culture where women and men faced with pregnancy decisions are transformed by the Gospel of Jesus Christ and empowered to choose life for their unborn children and abundant life for their families." Its mission statement is: "Acknowledging that every human life begins at conception and is worthy of protection, Care Net offers compassion, hope, and help to anyone considering abortion by presenting them with realistic alternatives and Christ-centered support through our life-affirming network of pregnancy centers, churches, organizations, and individuals."
23. S. L. Brown, "Marriage and Child Well-being: Research and Policy Perspectives," *Journal of Marriage and Family* 75.5 (Oct. 1, 2010): 1059–77, http://www.ncbi.nlm.nih.gov/pmc/articles/PMC3091824/#!po=40.6250; Gregory Acs and Sandi Nelson, "What Do 'I Do's Do? Potential Benefits of Marriage for Cohabiting Couples with Children," *New Federalism: National Survey of America's Families*, B-59 (2004): 1–7, http://www.urban.org/publications/311001.html.
24. L. B. Finer et al., "Reasons U.S. Women Have Abortions: Quantitative and Qualitative Perspectives," *Perspectives on Sexual Reproductive Health* 37.3 (September 2005): 110–08, doi:10.1363/psrh.37.110.05.
25. C. Coyle et al., "Inadequate Preabortion Counseling and Decision Conflict as Predictors of Subsequent Relationship Difficulties and Psychological Stress in Men and Women," *Traumatology* 16.1 (2010): 16–30, doi:10.1177/

15344765609347550; C. Coyle, "Men and Abortion: A Review of Empirical Reports," *Internet Journal of Mental Health*, 3.2 (2007), https://www.researchgate.net/publication/26453706_Men_and_Abortion_A_Review_of_Empirical_Reports_Concerning_the_Impact_of_Abortion_on_Men.

26. Guy Condon and David Hazard, *Fatherhood Aborted: The Profound Effects of Abortion on Men* (Carol Stream, IL: Tyndale House, 2001), introduction, xxv–xxvii.
27. *Pregnancy Centers Stand the Test of Time*, 16.
28. Ibid.
29. Ibid.
30. Ibid.

Chapter 20: The Pro-Life Movement: A Last Line of Protection for Black Women and Their Babies

1. Membership advertisement for the American Birth Control League, *Birth Control Review* 16.12 (December 1932), 319.
2. The language of "straighten it out" is that of Margaret Sanger. See "Letter from Margaret Sanger to Dr. C. J. Gamble," Genius, https://genius.com/Margaret-sanger-letter-from-margaret-sanger-to-dr-cj-gamble-annotated.
3. "Planned Parenthood Action Fund: The Full List of our 2020 Endorsements," Planned Parenthood, https://www.plannedparenthoodaction.org/2020-endorsements/full-list.
4. Julian Lewis, "Can the Negro Afford Birth Control? [1945]," in *Call and Response: Key Debates in African American Studies*, eds. Henry Louis Gates Jr., and Jennifer Burton (New York: W. W. Norton, 2011), 504–06, at 504–05.
5. Meili Powell, "Erma Clardy Craven (1918–1994)," Black Past, https://www.blackpast.org/african-american-history/clardy-craven-erma-1918-1994/.
6. Shaila Dewan, "Anti-Abortion Ads Split Atlanta," *The New York Times*, https://www.nytimes.com/2010/02/06/us/06abortion.html.
7. "Our History," Trust Black Women, https://trustblackwomen.org/our-roots.
8. Meghan Sorensen, "Loretta Ross, founder of the modern-day Reproductive Justice movement, speaks at Amherst college," *Daily Collegian*, https://dailycollegian.com/2019/10/loretta-ross-founder-of-the-modern-day-reproductive-justice-movement-speaks-at-amherst-college/.
9. Jill Stanek, "Inside Congressional Caucus Briefing on How to Block Pro-life Gains in Black Community," Jill Stanek, https://www.jillstanek.com/2012/05/inside-congressional-caucus-briefing-on-how-to-block-pro-life-gains-in-black-community/.
10. William McGurn, "White Supremacy and Abortion," *Wall Street Journal*, https://www.wsj.com/articles/white-supremacy-and-abortion-11567460392.
11. Stoyan Zaimov, "'Abortion Is Sacred, a Blessing, Life-Saving'? Controversial Billboard Campaign Launches in Ohio," The Christian Post, https://www.christianpost.com/news/abortion-is-sacred-a-blessing-life-saving-controversial-billboard-campaign-launches-in-ohio-212701/.

12. Ryan Bomberger, "Billboard Companies Promote Abortion But Censor Pro-life Messaging in Black Community," Townhall, https://townhall.com/columnists/ryanbomberger/2020/02/13/billboard-companies-promote-abortion-but-censor-prolife-messaging-in-black-community-n2561275 (emphasis in original).
13. "Fact Sheet," Planned Parenthood, https://www.plannedparenthood.org/files/8013/9611/6937/Opposition_Claims_About_Margaret_Sanger.pdf.
14. Ibid.
15. Ibid.
16. Imani Gandy, "How False Narratives of Margaret Sanger Are Being Used to Shame Black Women," August 20, 2015, Rewire News Group, https://rewirenewsgroup.com/article/2015/08/20/false-narratives-margaret-sanger-used-shame-black-women/.
17. Sarah Zagorski, "Black Feminist Tasha Fierce Brags: I Just Had an Abortion and Don't Regret It," LifeNews, https://www.lifenews.com/2015/01/13/black-feminist-tasha-fierce-brags-i-just-had-an-abortion-and-dont-regret-it/.
18. "Why pro-life is bad," Reddit, https://www.reddit.com/r/prochoice/comments/iup375/why_prolife_is_bad/_.
19. Justice Blackmun wrote: "The [state of Texas] argue[s] that the fetus is a 'person' within the language and meaning of the Fourteenth Amendment. In support of this, they outline at length and in detail the well-known facts of fetal development. If this suggestion of personhood is established, [Jane Roe's] case, of course, collapses, for the fetus' right to life would then be guaranteed specifically by the Amendment" (https://caselaw.findlaw.com/us-supreme-court/410/113.html). See chapter 6 in this volume by Joshua Craddock.
20. "Why pro-life is bad," Reddit, https://www.reddit.com/r/prochoice/comments/iup375/why_prolife_is_bad/.
21. Lauren Enriquez, "After Ralph Northam, the 'Bodily Autonomy' Argument for Abortion Is Shot," February 11, 2019, The Federalist, https://thefederalist.com/2019/02/11/ralph-northam-bodily-autonomy-argument-abortion-shot/.
22. "Black Lives Matter," Planned Parenthood Advocacy Fund of Massachusetts, Inc., https://www.plannedparenthoodaction.org/planned-parenthood-advocacy-fund-massachusetts-inc/black-lives-matter.
23. Save PPGNY, https://saveppgny.wordpress.com.
24. Samantha Schmidt, "Planned Parenthood to Remove Margaret Sanger's Name from N.Y. Clinic over Views on Eugenics," July 21, 2020, *The Washington Post*, https://www.washingtonpost.com/history/2020/07/21/margaret-sanger-planned-parenthood-eugenics/.
25. Darrah@PlannedParenthood, "Our Commitment to Black Communities," July 2, 2020, Planned Parenthood of the Pacific Southwest Blog, https://www.plannedparenthood.org/planned-parenthood-pacific-southwest/blog/our-commitment-to-black-communities (emphasis added).
26. "Rae Pickett, "A note from Paulette McElwain, our President and CEO," June 5, 2020, Virginia League for Planned Parenthood, https://www

.plannedparenthood.org/planned-parenthood-virginia-league/newsroom/a-note-from-paulette-mcelwain-our-president-and-ceo.

27. Jenna Tosh, "Central Coast Planned Parenthood confronts issues of race," August 1, 2020, *Santa Maria Times*, https://santamariatimes.com/opinion/columnists/jenna-tosh-central-coast-planned-parenthood-confronts-issues-of-race/article_d6abcf5e-b893-5bd5-9e69-cf9eebdff133.html.
28. "Black Lives Matter," Planned Parenthood Advocacy Fund of Massachusetts, Inc., https://www.plannedparenthoodaction.org/planned-parenthood-advocacy-fund-massachusetts-inc/black-lives-matter.
29. Cheryl Sullenger, "Video: 100 Women Hospitalized by Botched Abortions in 2019, Exposes the 'Safe Abortion' Lie" Operation Rescue, https://www.operationrescue.org/archives/video-100-women-hospitalized-by-botched-abortions-in-2019-exposes-the-safe-abortion-lie/.
30. Cheryl Sullenger, "Bleeding Abortion Patient Reveals Planned Parenthood's Safety Hazards Jumped the Mississippi River," December 31, 2019, Operation Rescue, https://www.operationrescue.org/archives/bleeding-abortion-patient-reveals-planned-parenthoods-safety-hazards-jumped-the-mississippi-river/.
31. Cheryl Sullenger, "80-Year Old Abortionist Keeps Working as Authorities Turn a Blind Eye to Her Abuses," Operation Rescue, https://www.operationrescue.org/archives/80-year-old-abortionist-keeps-working-as-authorities-turn-a-blind-eye-to-her-abuses/.
32. Cheryl Sullenger, "Morbelli Autopsy Report Does Not Address Carhart's Abandonment of Abortion Patient," May 30, 2013, Operation Rescue, https://www.operationrescue.org/archives/morbelli-autopsy-does-not-address-carharts-abandonment-of-abortion-patient/.
33. Gerard M. Nadal, "Abortion, Black Genocide, and The New Civil Rights Movement," Coming Home, https://gerardnadal.com/2011/01/13/abortion-black-genocide-and-the-new-civil-rights-movement/.
34. Ibid.
35. Lisa A. Maloney, "Pregnancy Care Centers Are Under Attack: HB 7070 is a Threat to Freedom of Speech and Religion," May 12, 2019, *The CT Mirror*, https://ctmirror.org/category/ct-viewpoints/pregnancy-care-centers-are-under-attack/.
36. Kathleen Megan, "Pitched Battle over Bill to Prohibit 'Deceptive Advertising' at Faith-based Pregnancy Centers," *The CT Mirror*, https://ctmirror.org/2019/02/11/pitched-battle-over-bill-to-prohibit-deceptive-advertising-at-faith-based-pregnancy-centers/.
37. https://www.protectingblacklife.org/.
38. "Frankly I had thought at the time Roe was decided, there was concern about population growth and particularly growth in populations that we don't want too many of" (Emily Bazelon, "The Place of Women on the Court," *The New York Times Mazazine*, https://www.nytimes.com/2009/07/12magazine/12ginsburg-t.html).